Vittorio Lingiardi, MD
Jack Drescher, MD
Editors

The Mental Health Professions and Homosexuality: International Perspectives

The Mental Health Professions and Homosexuality: International Perspectives has been co-published simultaneously as *Journal of Gay & Lesbian Psychotherapy*, Volume 7, Numbers 1/2 2003.

More pre-publication
REVIEWS, COMMENTARIES, EVALUATIONS . . .

"**E**XTRAORDINARY . . . Will support increased understanding of the international mental health community's training of and acceptance of gay and lesbian mental health processionals. Educators and practitioners will also be informed about what literature and research exists . . . on the experiences of gay and lesbian patients/clients with mental health care and psychotherapy. Gathering the thoughts and experiences of mental health practitioners and educators from different countries enriches the efforts being made to be more inclusive and understanding of diversity and, in particular, of sexual orientation and mental health."

Edward A. Wierzalis, PhD
Assistant Professor
Counselor Education
University of North Carolina
Charlotte

"**R**ICH IN HISTORICAL AND NARRATIVE DETAIL . . . provides an international perspective found in no other volume. INTERESTING AND INFORMATIVE. . . . Particularly unique and engaging are the descriptions of individuals who could be considered pioneers in the global mental health community and their efforts to effect more compassionate and competent treatment of gay and lesbian clients worldwide."

Kathleen Y. Ritter, PhD
Co-author
Handbook of Affirmative
Psychotherapy with Lesbians
and Gay Men
Professor
Counseling Psychology
California State University
at Bakersfield

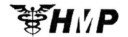

The Haworth Medical Press
An Imprint of The Haworth Press, Inc.

The Mental Health Professions and Homosexuality: International Perspectives

The Mental Health Professions and Homosexuality: International Perspectives has been co-published simultaneously as *Journal of Gay & Lesbian Psychotherapy*, Volume 7, Numbers 1/2 2003.

The *Journal of Gay & Lesbian Psychotherapy* Monographic "Separates"

Below is a list of "separates," which in serials librarianship means a special issue simultaneously published as a special journal issue or double-issue *and* as a "separate" hardbound monograph. (This is a format which we also call a "DocuSerial.")

"Separates" are published because specialized libraries or professionals may wish to purchase a specific thematic issue by itself in a format which can be separately cataloged and shelved, as opposed to purchasing the journal on an on-going basis. Faculty members may also more easily consider a "separate" for classroom adoption.

"Separates" are carefully classified separately with the major book jobbers so that the journal tie-in can be noted on new book order slips to avoid duplicate purchasing.

You may wish to visit Haworth's website at . . .

http://www.HaworthPress.com

. . . to search our online catalog for complete tables of contents of these separates and related publications.

You may also call 1-800-HAWORTH (outside US/Canada: 607-722-5857), or Fax: 1-800-895-0582 (outside US/Canada: 607-771-0012), or e-mail at:

getinfo@haworthpressinc.com

The Mental Health Professions and Homosexuality: International Perspectives, edited by Vittorio Lingiardi, MD, Jack Drescher, MD (Vol. 7, No. 1/2, 2003). *"PROVIDES A WORLDWIDE PERSPECTIVE that illuminates the psychiatric, psychoanalytic, and mental health professions' understanding and treatment of both lay and professional sexual minorities." (Bob Barrett, PhD, Professor and Counseling Program Coordinator, University of North Carolina at Charlotte)*

Sexual Conversion Therapy: Ethical, Clinical, and Research Perspectives, edited by Ariel Shidlo, PhD, Michael Schroeder, PsyD, and Jack Drescher, MD (Vol. 5, No. 3/4, 2001). *"THIS IS AN IMPORTANT BOOK. . . . AN INVALUABLE RESOURCES FOR MENTAL HEALTH PROVIDERS AND POLICYMAKERS. This book gives voice to those men and women who have experienced painful, degrading, and unsuccessful conversion therapy and survived. The ethics and misuses of conversion therapy practice are well documented, as are the harmful effects." (Joyce Hunter, DSW, Research Scientist, HIV Center for Clinical & Behavioral Studies, New York State Psychiatric Institute/Columbia University, New York City)*

Gay and Lesbian Parenting, edited by Deborah F. Glazer, PhD, and Jack Drescher, MD (Vol. 4, No. 3/4, 2001). *Richly textured, probing. These papers accomplish a rare feat: they explore in a candid, psychologically sophisticated, yet highly readable fashion how parenthood impacts lesbian and gay identity and how these identities affect the experience of parenting. Wonderfully informative. (Martin Stephen Frommer, PhD, Faculty/Supervisor, The Institute for Contemporary Psychotherapy, New York City).*

Addictions in the Gay and Lesbian Community, edited by Jeffrey R. Guss, MD, and Jack Drescher, MD (Vol. 3, No. 3/4, 2000). *Explores the unique clinical considerations involved in addiction treatment for gay men and lesbians, groups that reportedly use and abuse alcohol and substances at higher rates than the general population.*

The Mental Health Professions and Homosexuality: International Perspectives

Vittorio Lingiardi, MD
Jack Drescher, MD
Editors

The Mental Health Professions and Homosexuality: International Perspectives has been co-published simultaneously as *Journal of Gay & Lesbian Psychotherapy*, Volume 7, Numbers 1/2 2003.

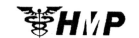

The Haworth Medical Press
An Imprint of
The Haworth Press, Inc.
New York • London • Oxford

Published by

The Haworth Medical Press®, 10 Alice Street, Binghamton, NY 13904-1580 USA

The Haworth Medical Press® is an imprint of The Haworth Press, Inc., 10 Alice Street, Binghamton, NY 13904-1580 USA.

The Mental Health Professions and Homosexuality: International Perspectives has been co-published simultaneously as *Journal of Gay & Lesbian Psychotherapy*, Volume 7, Numbers 1/2 2003.

Cover design by Lora Wiggins

Library of Congress Cataloging-in-Publication Data

Mental health professions and homosexuality : international perspectives / Vittorio Lingiardi, Jack Drescher, editors.
    p. ; cm.
    "Co-published simultaneously as Journal of gay & lesbian psychotherapy, Volume 7, Numbers 1/2, 2003."
    Includes bibliographical references and index.
    ISBN 0-7890-2058-0 (hard : alk. paper)–ISBN 0-7890-2059-9 (pbk. : alk. paper)
    1. Homosexuality. 2. Mental health personnel–Attitudes.
    [DNLM: 1. Attitude of Health Personnel. 2. Homosexuality–psychology. 3. Cross-Cultural Comparison. WM 62 M5487 2003] I. Lingiardi, Vittorio, 1960- II. Drescher, Jack, 1951- III. Journal of gay & lesbian psychotherapy.
  RC558.M47 2003
  616.85′83–dc21
                                        2002156760

Indexing, Abstracting & Website/Internet Coverage

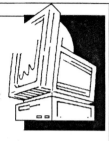

This section provides you with a list of major indexing & abstracting services. That is to say, each service began covering this periodical during the year noted in the right column. Most Websites which are listed below have indicated that they will either post, disseminate, compile, archive, cite or alert their own Website users with research-based content from this work. (This list is as current as the copyright date of this publication.)

(continued)

Special Bibliographic Notes related to special journal issues (separates) and indexing/abstracting:

- indexing/abstracting services in this list will also cover material in any "separate" that is co-published simultaneously with Haworth's special thematic journal issue or DocuSerial. Indexing/abstracting usually covers material at the article/chapter level.
- monographic co-editions are intended for either non-subscribers or libraries which intend to purchase a second copy for their circulating collections.
- monographic co-editions are reported to all jobbers/wholesalers/approval plans. The source journal is listed as the "series" to assist the prevention of duplicate purchasing in the same manner utilized for books-in-series.
- to facilitate user/access services all indexing/abstracting services are encouraged to utilize the co-indexing entry note indicated at the bottom of the first page of each article/chapter/contribution.
- this is intended to assist a library user of any reference tool (whether print, electronic, online, or CD-ROM) to locate the monographic version if the library has purchased this version but not a subscription to the source journal.
- individual articles/chapters in any Haworth publication are also available through the Haworth Document Delivery Service (HDDS).

The Mental Health Professions and Homosexuality: International Perspectives

CONTENTS

ABOUT THE EDITORS

Vittorio Lingiardi, MD, is Professor, Faculty of Psychology, University of Rome "La Sapienza." He has written numerous articles in Italian and international journals, has edited the Italian translations of numerous books on psychoanalysis, gender, and philosophy, and has authored five books in Italian, including *The Borderline Patient* (1990), *The Defense Mechanisms* (1994), *Personality Disorders* (1996), *Men in Love: Male Homosexualities from Ganymede to Batman* (1997, English Translation, 2002, Open Court, Chicago), and *The Personality Disordered Patient* (2001). Dr. Lingiardi, a member of the Editorial Board of the *Journal of Gay & Lesbian Psychotherapy*, is a psychiatrist and psychoanalyst affiliated with the International Association for Analytical Psychology (IAAP) and a member of the International Association for Relational Psychoanalysis and Psychotherapy (IAARP). He is in private practice in Milan, Italy.

Jack Drescher, MD, is a Fellow, Training and Supervising Analyst at the William Alanson White Psychoanalytic Institute and Clinical Assistant Professor of Psychiatry at SUNY–Brooklyn. He Chairs the Committee on Human Sexuality of the Group for the Advancement of Psychiatry (GAP) and Chairs the Committee on GLB Concerns of the American Psychiatric Association (APA). Author of *Psychoanalytic Therapy and the Gay Man* (1998, The Analytic Press), Dr. Drescher is in full time private practice in New York City.

As the World Turns: An Introduction

This special issue of the *Journal of Gay & Lesbian Psychotherapy* focuses on historical and contemporary attitudes of psychiatric, psychoanalytic and mental health professionals toward homosexuality in countries outside the United States. In the US, there has been a growing literature on the subject in the last two decades (see, for example, Lewes, 1988; Domenici and Lesser, 1995; Isay, 1996; Magee and Miller, 1997; Drescher, 1998; Group for the Advancement of Psychiatry, 2000; Shidlo, Schroeder and Drescher, 2001). However, there appears to be much less written in other countries. This collection is an attempt at beginning to correct that omission.

In soliciting contributors for this collection, international authors were asked to answer, as best as they could, three questions related to their own countries:

1. What are the prevailing theoretical models about homosexuality that can be found in the professional literature in your country?

2. What is known about the actual clinical experience of gay and lesbian individuals seeking help from psychiatric or other mental health professionals? This question has two parts:

    a. How does the professional literature talk about the subjective experiences of gay and lesbian patients/clients?

    b. What kinds of published reports or anecdotal tales are told about the experience of seeing a mental health provider who knows the patient is gay or lesbian?

3. What is the status of openly gay and lesbian mental health professionals in your country? How is the issue of being openly gay or lesbian talked about or is it talked about at all? Where there is no published literature, anecdotes are acceptable.

[Haworth co-indexing entry note]: "As the World Turns: An Introduction." Lingiardi, Vittorio, and Jack Drescher. Co-published simultaneously in *Journal of Gay & Lesbian Psychotherapy* (The Haworth Medical Press, an imprint of The Haworth Press, Inc.) Vol. 7, No. 1/2, 2003, pp. 1-6; and: *The Mental Health Professions and Homosexuality: International Perspectives* (ed: Vittorio Lingiardi, and Jack Drescher) The Haworth Medical Press, an imprint of The Haworth Press, Inc., 2003, pp. 1-6. Single or multiple copies of this article are available for a fee from The Haworth Document Delivery Service [1-800-HAWORTH, 9:00 a.m. - 5:00 p.m. (EST). E-mail address: getinfo@haworthpressinc.com].

10.1300/J236v07n01_01

The searching, collecting and editing of the contributions that compose this volume have made for a fascinating and deeply relational experience. Never has the definition of the computer being "a box that contains other people" (Stone, 1995, p. 28) been as appropriate as in this case. This project would have been unthinkable without the help of e-mail and on-line research. In the last couple of years, the editors feel that they have become a part of a truly international and collaborative community. From Italy to Finland, from the United States to India, this volume represents a living web of reports and narratives. The most extraordinary aspect of this network is its capacity to connect, in a "global" way, a diverse range of "non-global" or local realities.

Of course, this collection only focuses on a small portion of a potentially infinite number of experiences and realities. And not just because the world is really so big, but also because each culture has created, over time, different ways to look at homosexual people and different ways to include or exclude them from social and public health policies. As we put "the homosexualities" in front of the mirror of local cultures, the effect obtained is one of amplification and multiplication (see Murray, 2000; Lingiardi, 2002). Thus the editors had to make some choices. It was only possible to cover, for space reasons, a few geographical and cultural areas.

However, space limitations were not the only reason some territories remain unexplored. There is another reason, having nothing to do with the vastness of the topic, but with the difficulty in getting information from many parts of the world. Some countries, indeed whole continents, were silent; others may have spoken to us, but the dialogue was insufficient to generate a coherent narrative. For example, in soliciting a contribution from a gay psychiatrist in Argentina, he eventually responded:

> I'm sorry to say that my answer is "no." In fact, I'm not able to write a proper and serious paper on the subject you need. I'm an outsider in Argentina . . . So, I have no exchange with colleagues about homosexuality; there are no rules. We don't have any literature or reports. Everything is closed. There is a very small group of openly gay therapists, but they are not relevant in the milieu. Of course, I know some things and how some people think . . . I don't want to write a paper based on gossip. I cannot base my article on nothing but my own word because then I'll be gossiping too. I'm really sorry. I've many things to chat [about] but nothing to write. I want to thank you for your invitation and I lament living in a very fascist country.

Before making the e-mail acquaintance of Suresh Parekh, whose paper on India eventually found its way into this volume, the following letter came from the famous Indian psychiatrist and psychoanalyst, Sudhir Kakar (1990):

Thank you for your e-mail. Alas, I have no idea of how mental health professionals in India look at gay issues. A result of my almost non-existent contacts with the psychiatric community and a total absence of the topic in the Indian psychiatric literature (which in itself is an important comment but not too useful for your purpose). Thus my regrets.

Similar responses were received from Russia. It was even more difficult to get in touch with mental health professionals from Islamic countries. Although not entirely surprised by the difficulties in countries where homosexuality is illegal and persecuted, the chain of refusals received from French colleagues, many of them affiliated with the International Psychoanalytic Association, was astonishing. Some, for example, gave a strong impression that they believed the issue of gay and lesbian analysts is a "political" (and therefore non-analytic) issue and an "American problem" having no relevance to European societies.

The papers that ultimately made their way into this volume give some idea of the distance that has been traveled in order for mental health professionals to arrive at a non-discriminating attitude towards gay and lesbian people. But, as noted above, contained in this volume is only the speaking part of the world. In a future thematic volume, hopefully in the near future, the editors would like to give a voice to the continents not represented here: Africa, Australia, and South America.

The first part of this volume is from European contributors. Daniel Twomey describes "British Psychoanalytic Attitudes Towards Homosexuality" from the beginning of the twentieth century to the present. Particular attention is paid in his paper to the evolution of theoretical and clinical models in the United Kingdom. He cautiously notes that even though a non-pathologizing attitude seems to be prevailing, the criteria for acceptance of openly gay and lesbian candidates for psychoanalytic training remains a thorny and embarrassing question. He also addresses some of the changing views within British psychiatry as well.

In "From Perversion to Sexual Identity: Concepts of Homosexuality and Its Treatment in Germany," Falk Stakelbeck and Udo Frank focus on the evolution of mental health professional attitudes in their country. Notwithstanding a prevailing non-pathologizing attitude, the German scientific community has produced very few empirical studies. Stakelbeck and Frank's paper is the first to report on three surveys of German psychoanalytic institutes regarding their admission policies toward gay and lesbian applicants and candidates. They also include previously unpublished data showing changes in institute policies.

As we find in Udo Rauchfleisch's "Psychiatric, Psychoanalytic, and Mental Health Profession Attitudes Toward Homosexuality in Switzerland," the situation is not very different than in Germany. In Switzerland, however, lesbian and gay therapists seem more organized: they work together in informal groups and have a national organization. But, as elsewhere in Europe, Swiss psychoanalytic institutes are reluctant to accept gay and lesbian candidates.

For many German and Swiss psychiatrists and psychoanalysts, the work of Fritz Morgenthaler, MD (1919-1984)–a Middle-European intellectual outsider who formulated a psychoanalytic conception of a non-pathological homosexuality–has been very influential. For this reason, this volume concludes with Luisa Mantovani's interview of Paul Parin, MD, an 85 year old collaborator, colleague, and friend of Morgenthaler.

Moving to Northern Europe and the Scandinavian peninsula, presented next are Reidar Kjær's "Look to Norway? Gay Issues and Mental Health Across the Atlantic Ocean" and Olli Stålström and Jussi Nissinen's "Homosexuality in Finland: The Decline of Psychoanalysis' Illness Model of Homosexuality." The authors describe the influence of European and American theoretical models in Scandinavia and–notwithstanding increasing social tolerance of homosexuality and increased expansion of gay and lesbian civil rights–they underscore the lack of indigenous mental health research about homosexuality.

The "Italian case" is taken up by Paola Capozzi and Vittorio Lingiardi's "Happy Italy? The Mediterranean Experience of Homosexuality, Psychoanalysis and the Mental Health Professions." Outlining the social, religious and cultural story of homosexuality in their country, the authors focus their attention on the typical "Italian" situation of "don't ask-don't tell." They offer a detailed review of the Italian scientific literature from 1930 to the present, concluding that only in the last ten years has the Italian mental health community started to come to terms with its own antihomosexual biases.

The second part of this collection is dedicated to the two biggest Asian countries: China and India. In "From 'Long Yang' and 'Dui Shi' to Tongzhi," Jin Wu describes how homosexuality was fairly tolerated, although not entirely accepted, in ancient China. It is interesting to know that a pathological view of homosexuality was "imported" by the Chinese from Western civilizations. The 2001 Chinese Classification of Mental Disorders (CCMD-3) removed the diagnosis of homosexuality, but the tongzhi (gay) community in China has much work left to do before achieving full civil rights.

As Suresh Parekh states in his hopeful title, "Homosexuality in India: The Light at the End of the Tunnel," as in China, the pre-modern times of Hindu civilization seemed more tolerant of same-sex relationships. In the second part of his paper, Parekh discusses the changing attitude toward gays and lesbians, their legal status and the emergence of gay and lesbian civil rights organizations in modern India. Because Indian psychological and psychiatric literature regarding homosexuality is very scarce, the author presents anecdotes, unpublished reports and articles from gay magazines to give some sense of the situation in that country.

The third section of this volume is dedicated to international, mental health organizations from the perspectives of two insiders. In "The Emergence of an International Lesbian, Gay, and Bisexual Psychiatric Movement," Gene Nakajima tells the story of organizational efforts slowly developing outside of North America. Changes are taking place in both the World Psychiatric Association, and elsewhere, with the help of the Association of Gay and Lesbian Psychiatrists (AGLP). Although only seven percent of AGLP is made up of psychiatrists outside the US and Canada, its members have helped intervene in depathologizing homosexuality in both Japan and China. They are also working to eliminate the diagnosis of egodystonic sexual orientation in the World Health Organization's *International Classification of Diseases* (ICD-10).

Ralph Roughton (2001a, 2001b) is a leading figure in helping the American Psychoanalytic Association rethink its historical positions on homosexuality. He provides a first-person account of his experience with "The International Psychoanalytical Association and Homosexuality." Both Nakajima and Roughton's accounts are a testament to the power of committed individuals to effect important social changes.

Vittorio Lingiardi, MD
Jack Drescher, MD

REFERENCES

Domenici, T. & Lesser, R. C., eds. (1995), *Disorienting Sexuality: Psychoanalytic Reappraisals of Sexual Identities*. New York: Routledge.

Drescher, J. (1998), *Psychoanalytic Therapy and the Gay Man*. Hillsdale, NJ: The Analytic Press.

Group for the Advancement of Psychiatry (2000), *Homosexuality and the Mental Health Professions: The Impact of Bias*. Hillsdale, NJ: The Analytic Press.

Isay, R. (1996), *Becoming Gay: The Journey to Self-Acceptance*. New York: Pantheon.

Kakar, S. (1990), *Intimate Relations: Exploring Indian Sexuality*. Chicago: University of Chicago Press.

Lewes, K. (1988), *The Psychoanalytic Theory of Male Homosexuality*. New York: Simon and Schuster. Reissued as *Psychoanalysis and Male Homosexuality* (1995), Northvale, NJ: Aronson.

Lingiardi, V. (2002), *Men in Love: Male Homosexualities from Ganymede to Batman*. Chicago: Open Court.

Magee, M. & Miller, D. (1997), *Lesbian Lives: Psychoanalytic Narratives Old and New*. Hillsdale, NJ: The Analytic Press.

Murray, S. O. (2000), *Homosexualities*. Chicago: The University of Chicago Press.

Roughton, R. (2001a), Dialogue: Homosexuality: Clinical and Technical Issues. *International Psychoanalysis: Newsletter of the IPA*, 10(1): 17-19.

Roughton, R. (2001b), Four Men in Treatment. *J. Amer. Psychoanal. Assn.*, 49(4): 187-1218.

Shidlo, A., Schroeder, M. & Drescher, J., eds. (2001), *Sexual Conversion Therapy: Ethical, Clinical and Research Perspectives.* New York: The Haworth Medical Press.

Stone, A. R. (1995), *The War of Desire and Technology at the Close of the Mechanical Age.* Boston, MA: MIT Press.

British Psychoanalytic Attitudes Towards Homosexuality

Daniel Twomey, DSW

SUMMARY. This paper describes the attitudes of British Psychoanalysis toward homosexuality, starting from the time of Ernest Jones to the present day. It traces the development of psychoanalytic theory from its total pathologising of all expressions of homosexuality towards a more questioning and non-pathologising formulation. The article illustrates how changes in psychoanalytic theory and practice both mirror and are influenced by the changing legal and societal status of homosexuality in the United Kingdom. Although openly gay and lesbian candidates are beginning to be accepted into psychoanalytic training, the continued existence of antihomosexual prejudice and bias suggest an ongoing need for continuing education and concern. *[Article copies available for a fee from The Haworth Document Delivery Service: 1-800-HAWORTH. E-mail address: <getinfo@haworthpressinc.com> Website: <http://www.HaworthPress. com>* © 2003 by The Haworth Press, Inc. All rights reserved.]

KEYWORDS. British psychiatry, British psychoanalysis, gay and lesbian candidates, homosexuality, psychoanalytic training, psychopathology

Daniel Twomey is a member of the British Association of Psychotherapists, Chair of the Psychoanalytic Section and Vice Chair of the Council. He is in private practice in North London.

The author wishes to thank Mary Lynne Ellis and Lucia Asnaghi for their support while writing this paper.

[Haworth co-indexing entry note]: "British Psychoanalytic Attitudes Towards Homosexuality." Twomey, Daniel. Co-published simultaneously in *Journal of Gay & Lesbian Psychotherapy* (The Haworth Medical Press, an imprint of The Haworth Press, Inc.) Vol. 7, No. 1/2, 2003, pp. 7-22; and: *The Mental Health Professions and Homosexuality: International Perspectives* (ed: Vittorio Lingiardi, and Jack Drescher) The Haworth Medical Press, an imprint of The Haworth Press, Inc., 2003, pp. 7-22. Single or multiple copies of this article are available for a fee from The Haworth Document Delivery Service [1-800-HAWORTH, 9:00 a.m. - 5:00 p.m. (EST). E-mail address: getinfo@haworthpressinc.com].

10.1300/J236v07n01_02

There has been an increasingly tolerant social and political attitude in the United Kingdom towards gays and lesbians. This was illustrated recently in the reality TV show, "Big Brother," where an openly gay man was voted the winner by millions of viewers. The UK now has an equal age of consent; gay people are accepted in the armed forces and openly gay members of parliament occupy positions in the government. The present Labour government is proposing a new law, which would make discrimination illegal in employment and training on the basis of age, sexual orientation and religion.

These societal and political changes have brought a change in theorising and official policy with regards to accepting gay and lesbian candidates for training. There are two registration bodies for psychotherapists in the UK: the British Confederation of Psychotherapists (BCP) and the United Kingdom Conference for Psychotherapy (UKCP). Nearly all training bodies belonging to these organisations have an Equal Opportunity Policy, which states that "they do not discriminate on grounds of sexual orientation." This is indeed progress; however, as this paper will detail, there is still some cause for concern.

In a recent study published in the *British Journal of Psychiatry* (Bartlett, Philips and King, 2001), among a sample of 218 members of the British Confederation of Psychotherapists, 64% believed that a gay or lesbian client's "sexual orientation was central to their difficulties." The study's authors further concluded that "Gays and lesbians seeking psychoanalysis or psychotherapy in the National Health Service (NHS) or outside it for personal and/or training purposes will be unlikely to find a gay or lesbian therapist if they want one. The British Confederation of Psychotherapists' practitioners takes on gay and lesbian clients/patients, although many do not see these social identities as relevant to the therapeutic process. Evidence from this study indicates that such clients/patients may encounter overt or covert bias, including the pathologisation of homosexuality per se."

HISTORIC PSYCHOANALYTIC THEORY AND PRACTICE

As far as I have been able to ascertain there are no "out" gay psychoanalysts in the UK. Furthermore, in my extensive research for this paper, I was unable to find any British psychoanalyst who was of the theoretical belief that homosexuality could be a normal, healthy end-point of psychosexual development. These attitudes among psychoanalytically-oriented psychotherapists could be traced back to Ernest Jones, the psychiatrist who founded the British Institute of Psychoanalysis in 1919. In 1921, he requested an opinion as to whether a "homosexual" candidate should be accepted for analytic training. He received the following reply in a *Circular Letter* from Freud and Otto Rank (1921):

"We do not want to exclude such persons because we cannot condone their legal prosecution, we believe that a decision in such cases should be reserved for an examination of the individuals other qualities" (quoted in Lewes, 1988, p. 33). If this advice had been accepted, the relationship between British psychoanalysis and the gay and lesbian community may have been very different from the one that eventually developed. Jones rejected their advice because he believed that "homosexuals" were fixated at an early stage of development, i.e., they had not resolved the Oedipus complex. Thus homosexual men and lesbians were excluded from psychoanalytic training and all "homosexuals" were pathologised.

In the ensuing years, many comments of British psychoanalysts and the language they used to describe homosexuality and "homosexuals" illustrated a deep level of antihomosexual bias. Ronald Fairbairn (1946), for example, was one of the most important theorists of British object relations theory.[1] He recommended that "homosexuals" should not be offered psychotherapy since they did not want "cure but re-instatement" (p. 293). He also thought that they should be removed from society and placed in settlement camps (p. 294). Michael Balint (1956), considered by many to be Ferenczi's successor, came to England from Hungary in 1939 and joined the British Analytic Society. He classified homosexuality as a perversion because "of the atmosphere of pretence[2] and denial that is so characteristic of this group of perversions" (p. 24) He also believed that "without normal intercourse there is no real contentment" (p. 24).

Ismond Rosen,[3] a member of the British Psychoanalytic Society (BPAS), edited a book entitled *Sexual Deviation*. In the introduction, homosexuality is linked to a wide range of sexual disorders: "Sexual deviations are usually separated into categories according to the predominant and outstanding behaviour. These categories include homosexuality, sexual activities with immature partners of sex (paedophilia), dead people (necrophilia), animals (bestiality), or inanimate objects (fetishism). Also included are sado-masochism, sexual violence, rape, incest, exhibitionism, voyeurism, and transexualism" (Rosen, 1979, p. 3).[4]

These views could be dismissed as old-fashioned; however, they still resonate with more recent statements by British analysts. Peter Hildebrand, another training analyst of the BPAS who also worked at the Tavistock clinic, wrote in 1992, "aspects of the homosexual lifestyle are profoundly unacceptable to non homosexuals" (p. 457) and that "The often hidden desire to harm the other person, is central to all forms of sexual perversion whether sado-masochism fetishist or homosexual" (p. 458). In a criticism of the work of the hospices and voluntary bodies caring for people with AIDS, he further added, "The difference between the psychoanalytic approach and the approach of the caring organisations which I have described is that we *do not allow* for a collusion that they ["homosexuals"] are living a sanctified life in the way in which the hospice group do and we would, in fact, *insist* very strongly on the profound aggression towards the object which seems central to their psychopathology" (1992, p. 459).

Returning to the early psychoanalytic years, among the individuals whose theoretical work is most representative of mainstream British theorizing about homosexuality are Glover, Anna Freud, the Kleinian school, Gillespie, Glasser, and Limentani. Edward Glover was born, in 1888, into a strict Presbyterian background and became a powerful member of the British Society, second only to Jones. He maintained that homosexuality was a perversion "being a regression to an earlier stage of sexual development, (but was) the most advanced and organised form of sexual perversion" (1939, p. 257). Nevertheless, Glover held out the possibility for a non-pathological form of homosexual relatedness and a non-neurotic group of homosexuals: "the manifestations of homosexual love-feelings and the attitude to the love object cannot be distinguished from those associated with normal heterosexual love" (1939, p. 257). Years later, he wrote "Some analysts have maintained that every homosexual presents signs of neurosis. This is certainly not true of the homosexual group as a whole" (1960, p. 212). Glover campaigned, in the tradition of Freud, for the decriminalisation of homosexual acts. Glover, William Gillespie, Wilfred Bion and Hannah Segal had a powerful influence on The Wolfenden Commission, which led to the 1967 legalisation of homosexuality in the UK. However, they all considered homosexuality a perversion and supported the ban on admitting gay and lesbian candidates into psychoanalytic training.

Anna Freud had a very different view from her father in that she saw homosexuality as an illness that could be cured. She formulated her theories from her analysis of four homosexual men. She postulated that "homosexuals" had lost their masculinity and attempted to regain it through identification with their partners. Men who choose a passive partner vicariously enjoyed a passive or receptive mode, whilst men who preferred an active partner recovered their lost masculinity (1949, p. 96). That masculinity had once been there and had gotten lost was a new theoretical contribution. In analysing homosexual men, Anna Freud recommended interpreting the transference between the same-sex partners rather than the transference between the analyst and the patient (1952). Like modern-day reparative therapists, she admonished her homosexual patients not to "act out" their sexuality if they wished to get the benefit of treatment (1954).

Melanie Klein theorised that the mechanisms operating in paranoia enter "into every homosexual activity" and felt "The sexual act between men always, in part, serves to satisfy sadistic impulses" (1932, p. 262). The Kleinian analyst Rosenfeld (1949), in a reversal of Freud's (1911) formulation of the Schreber case, saw homosexuality as a defence against paranoia. Hannah Segal (1990), the leading Kleinian in the UK today, is known to be opposed to homosexuals becoming parents and sees all homosexuality as an attack on the heterosexual couple.

William Gillespie was analysed in Vienna by Edward Hirshmann and joined the BPAS in 1932. He had influence in both British and international psychoanalysis, discarded Freud's bisexuality theory, and regarded all expressions of homosexuality as a sign of disturbance. Gillespie hypothesised two categories of homosexual behaviour: one as a preoedipal fixation, the other as a regressive defence against oedipal problems (1964).

Mervin Glasser (1977) a training analyst in the BPAS, and a strong influence on British theorising about homosexuality, said that "homosexual men behaved histrionically and gave the gay behaviour of homosexuals its apt name." He also said that "the homosexual's" ability "to live a part rather than to merely play it" was reminiscent of "psychopathy." Glasser also maintained that women became lesbians "because of the persistence of the attempt to deny what they believe to be their anatomical inferiority." In the "Core complex" (1979), he postulates a universal stage of development. The need to engage intimately, to fuse with another is in conflict–because of the terror of engulfment it arouses–with the need to withdraw from and to destroy the object with which it wishes to fuse. The prototypical object is the mother. This withdrawal leads to feelings of abandonment. In order to compensate for this loneliness, the subject begins to re-desire fusion. Glasser held that all the "homosexuals" he had known sexualised the aggression with the mother and converted it into sadism, thus setting up a sadomasochistic relationship with the mother which generalises to all their other relationships. This theory has been applied extensively to the treatment of "homosexuals" in England, and underlies the psychoanalytic assertion that all gays are promiscuous, sado-masochistic and incapable of loving and lasting relationships.[5]

In line with Stoller's belief that (1985, p. 97) "It is better to talk of the homosexualities rather than a homosexuality," British Psychoanalyst Adam Limentani (1979) proposed three classifications of homosexuality. However, none of them allowed for the possibility of an ordinary, non-pathological homosexual development:

1. Situational homosexuality, as in prisons, which is no longer acted upon when the individual returns to ordinary life.
2. A homosexuality based on a fear of castration and which is amenable to psychoanalytic intervention.
3. A homosexuality which is a defence against psychosis and which is not amenable to psychotherapy without involving grave risks.

Eric Rayner (1990), a training analyst at the BPAS, in his book on *Human Development*, describes homosexuality as "a perversion and a dislike of the idea of the penis within a vagina." He also states that because the biological urge to recreate has been diverted, "Something psychologically very intense must be happening" This book is still used on many social work and counselling courses.

In 1985, the French analyst, Janine Chasseguet-Smirgel, became the Freud Memorial Professor at the University of London. Although she is not British, she has had a very strong influence on British psychoanalytic theorising on homosexuality. She maintains that all homosexuality is pathological and perverted: "Their ['homosexuals'] tendency to organise themselves and to claim public approval helps many individuals to consider their perversion not as an illness but as a different or even superior form of human existence" (1985b, p. 90). Repeatedly referring to "homosexuals" as "perverts," Chasseguet-Smirgel further maintains that the creative works of "perverts" are only "pseudocreative"; for example, she dismisses Oscar Wilde's work as being only of a "glitzy" creativity . . . The work of art achieved by subjects presenting such a structural chore [perverts] and however original it claims to be is nevertheless nothing but an imitation" (p. 71).

Today, attitudes like these in the UK have had an impact on decisions regarding who can and cannot train as a psychoanalyst. There are only three papers in English which theoretically argue that certain "homosexuals," like certain heterosexuals, are suitable to undergo intensive psychoanalytic training (Cunningham, 1991; Ellis, 1994; Mendoza, 1997). And although it is becoming increasingly difficult to discriminate on the basis of sexual orientation in the UK, anecdotal accounts indicate that psychoanalysts and psychoanalytic psychotherapists may be nevertheless practising antigay discrimination.[6]

PROTEST AND REFORM

It is crucial to understand that homosexuality in the UK was only decriminalised in 1967. Many gay men entrapped by police ended up at the Portman clinic where many of the psychoanalytic theoreticians who are cited above worked. Theories formulated up to 1967 unequivocally mirrored societal feelings about homosexuality; as Drescher (1995) puts it "it is extremely difficult to separate a scientific theory from the cultural matrix in which theories are formulated" (p. 240). As a result, most of the theories cited above were developed from the analysis and psychotherapy of "homosexuals" who sought treatment because of criminal sanctions against homosexuality or who had been sent for treatment by the courts. Therefore, during this time, accepting an openly gay man for psychoanalytic training, or one who was in a gay partnership, was tantamount to accepting someone who was involved in criminal activity.

The first recorded protest in England against laws that criminalised and theories that pathologised homosexuals took place in Highbury Fields London in

1950. A group of gays met and chanted "One-two-five-six-eight! Gay is as good as straight!" It would take another thirty years before a group of gay psychotherapists publicly challenged psychoanalytic theories of homosexuality. This challenge took place in the 1980s at a public lecture given by Ismond Rosen at University College London. A group of gay and lesbian psychotherapists in the audience, organized by PACE, asked questions and put forward ideas which challenged the belief that all homosexuality was pathological (PACE, Project for Advice and Education, is a counselling psychotherapy and community work organization for lesbian and gay men).

In 1995, the next and more significant protest against the pathological model took place when the Association for Psychoanalytic Psychotherapy in the National Health invited Charles Socarides to give their annual lecture. Ismond Rosen was the discussant. Since both speakers viewed homosexuality as pathological, the failure of the association to provide a speaker who would put forward a different theoretical viewpoint caused concern. At a meeting of Psychotherapists and Counsellors for Social Responsibility, Andrew Samuels, a Jungian training analyst, and Joanna Ryan, a psychoanalytic psychotherapist, decided to respond to Socarides' visit. They together with Mary Lynne Ellis organised a letter protesting the failure to provide a speaker with a different viewpoint. The letter was signed by 200 psychotherapists and became a "rallying point for many who worried about psychoanalytic theorising of homosexuality and its implication for practice" (Ellis, 1997).

Socarides' visit galvanised a group of psychotherapists, both gay and heterosexual, who were unwilling to accept theories that pathologised all expressions of homosexuality. They were instrumental in the national press eventually taking up the theoretical debate (Kogbara, 1995) and in organising in 1997 a conference in Cambridge on "Homosexuality and Psychoanalysis." Most of the speakers at the conference were gay or lesbian and 375 people attended.

Socarides' visit also polarised opinion against the British institute of Psychoanalysis which was labeled "homophobic" by the protest organisers. On the other side, according to one anecdotal report, the protesters were described as "fearing their identity will be destroyed and [people] who attack truth and free speech." This subsequent polarisation around this issue has had an adverse effect on scientific and intellectual debate about homosexuality in the UK. For example, only 6 members of the British Confederation of Psychotherapists attended the conference in Cambridge. Even today, efforts to have a public debate with psychoanalysts about their theoretical beliefs are proving more difficult, if not impossible to arrange. Christopher Shelly was unable to find a British psychoanalyst willing to write the chapter on *Psychoanalysis and Male Homosexuality* in his edited book *Contemporary Perspectives on Psychotherapy and Homosexualities* (1998).

Although they have withdrawn from the public arena, a private debate did take place within the BPAS. Some of the papers presented in this debate were published in the Society's bulletin, a publication only available to Society members. In preparing this paper for the *Journal of Gay & Lesbian Psychotherapy*, attempts were made to ascertain if any papers on homosexuality were written by members of the BPAS or the Society of Analytic Psychology in the last ten years. The librarians of both organisations found that none were written by members of the Society of Analytic Psychology while seven papers had appeared in the bulletin of the BPAS between 1996 and 1997. As a non-member of the BPAS, however, one had to apply to the librarian for permission to read the papers; this was granted in the case of 5 of the 7 papers.[7] Access was given on condition "that these papers are strictly not to be circulated beyond the named recipient–Daniel Twomey." In any event, permission was not granted to quote any part of the papers. It is not clear why the papers are being treated with such secrecy. It is worth noting, however, that a spirit of inquiry free from antihomosexual bias permeates the papers. Throughout the collection there exists a spirit of openness to new ideas, a willingness to rethink past assumptions, and a recognition that some of the samples used to generate theory in the past might not have been representative of the gay population.

There are other signs that psychoanalysts are gradually changing their thinking on homosexuality. In the current volume of the *British Journal of Psychotherapy*, Ann Zachary (2001), a psychoanalyst and psychiatrist, has written a paper, "Uneasy Triangles: A Brief Overview Of The History Of Homosexuality." The author accepts the universality of bisexuality. What she calls the triangles of (sin crime illness) (reaction resistance projection) and (mother child father) are useful in preventing discussions about homosexuality from becoming "polarised into two dimensional debate" about what is pathological and non-pathological. Zachary sees the Oedipus complex as dynamic and being negotiated internally throughout life. Zachary comments on the change "in our ability to challenge previously fixed polarisations such as heterosexuality and homosexuality and in recognising different sexualities." She goes on to suggest "that there will always be some sin, some crime and some illness for homosexuals and heterosexuals and that the answer lies in keeping things fluid and open minded not rigidly set in polarised positions." Another psychoanalyst, Sira Dermen, is quoted as saying in a lecture at Regents College London that "heterosexuality and homosexuality are solutions to anxiety-driven situations of which Oedipus remains paramount. Both are achievements in the technical sense.

The exclusion of gays and lesbians from psychoanalytic training was taken up in the British press in 1994. This public airing of the issue was stimulated by the work of Mary Lynne Ellis (1994) who researched both attitudes and policies of the main psychoanalytic training bodies with regard to the acceptance of gay and lesbian candidates. She reported encountering evasions, confusion and a reluctance to even discuss the issue among the organisations she interviewed. She was told by the Chair of Admissions at the Institute of Psychoanalysis that they "wondered about a homosexual's ability to work intensively with a lot of issues of a heterosexual nature such as relationships with children" (p. 511). He further went on to say "that they would worry if someone had made a firm choice of homosexuality as their sexual orientation and didn't feel that was something that needed to be considered in their lives" and he also believed that "a person's sexual adjustment would coincide with a heterosexual orientation" (p. 512). The British Association of Psychotherapists declined to give Ellis an interview, stating that her research "was not relevant to the selection policy of the BAP" (p. 514).

One gay analysand in training with another organisation told Ellis he had been told by his psychoanalyst "that if a report was required for assessment purposes, he could only respond negatively" adding that "Homosexuals can't be psychotherapists"(p. 513) while another psychoanalyst told a lesbian applicant that she would not be accepted for training at his institute because it was felt that she would be "insensitive to certain aspects of human relationships" (p. 513). These responses were consistent with a history of excluding of gay men and lesbians from psychoanalytic training which began with Jones and was later supported by Melanie Klein and Anna Freud.[8] After the British press took up the issue, journalist Paula Webb (1994) concluded that "Prejudice against homosexuality is as important for Gays and Lesbians on the couch as for those behind it."

In other words, there is no doubt that until very recently, there was a ban on accepting gays and lesbians for psychoanalytic training in the UK. That it operated unofficially–while being officially denied in public–is also verifiable. A qualitative study by Phillips, Bartlett, and King (2001, p. 80) found in a sample of 15 British Confederation of Psychotherapists members that their responses to the suggestion of having gay and lesbian trainees divided into two groups: (1) "those who were in full agreement with the current process of selection (for training) including the exclusion of gay and lesbians on the grounds of their sexuality; and (2) those who felt that current selection methods and criteria regarding gay and lesbians are inappropriate and outdated." That there is a change in British psychoanalysis is beyond doubt. The beginning of accepting openly gay and lesbian candidates into training has taken place. Attempts at building a non-pathological theory of homosexuality are being taken seriously. Equal access to training is soon to be enshrined in law.[9] In all likelihood, as in the United States, a greater change will only occur when gay and lesbian psychoanalysts come out of the "closet" and write and theorise about their own life work and sexuality.

PSYCHOANALYTIC PSYCHOTHERAPISTS

Today, members of the British Confederation of Psychotherapists now officially admit gay and lesbian trainees. In contrast to psychoanalysts, there have been many publications by psychoanalytic psychotherapists that are more accepting of gay and lesbian subjectivities. Many of these publications have appeared in *The British Journal of Psychotherapy*. In 1991, an author writing in that journal under the pseudonym of R. Cunningham[10] used a Kleinian approach to argue for the existence of a non-pathological form of homosexuality. In contrast to traditional Kleinian theory, she said many "homosexuals" are capable of achieving the depressive position and have the ability to appreciate the "beauty and creativity" of the heterosexual couple in reproductive sexual intercourse.

In 1993, Noreen O'Connor and Joanna Ryan's *Wild Desires and Mistaken Identities* was published. The authors argued for "the need to create a theoretical and conceptual space for non pathological possibilities in relation to homosexuality" (p. 10). They called for clinicians to pay more attention to their countertransference responses when formulating theories and they note "the absence of counter-transference considerations in case studies describing work with homosexual patients" (p. 11).[11] They suggested an equivalence in theorising between heterosexuality and homosexuality, allowing for pathological and non pathological variations of both, which "would greatly advance psychoanalytic understanding of homosexuality in its many forms" (p. 11). Susannah Izzard's paper *Oedipus-Baby and Bath Water?* (1999) enters the debate between some who would abolish the Oedipus complex from psychoanalytic theory, others who would deconstruct it like O'Connor and Ryan (1993), and those who would reform it. Izzard, like the Americans Isay (1996) and Lewes (1988), favours reformation by keeping the oedipal baby and meeting him afresh.

David Jones' (2001) "Shame, Disgust, Anger and Revenge" pleads for more insights into homosexuality and a treatment of "homosexuals" derived from an examination of one's countertransference toward them. Steven Mendoza's (2001) "Genital and Phallic Homosexuality" argues that it is the quantity of genital or phallic organisation involved in a sexual relationship which determines its psychological maturity: "Sexual orientation does not determine or even, to a reliable, extent, indicate, any special disturbance requiring particular treatment . . . A homosexual, limited to his or her own sex, may be capable of a love of the other in the sense of a whole object which may be called genital" (p. 155).

ANALYTICAL PSYCHOLOGY

As Andrew Samuels[12] (1985) notes, homosexuality has not received much attention from Jungians. However, it is common knowledge that for many years, numerous members of London's Society of Analytical Psychology have accepted and taught non-pathological views on homosexuality. In contrast to Hildebrand (1992), Jungian writers have demonstrated a deep level of non-pathologising empathy and understanding towards people afflicted with AIDS. As Frantz (1995) notes, ". . . it is no longer them it is now us" (p. 257) and "The trauma experienced by the psyche in AIDS is beyond the ability to articulate of anyone who does not have the disease. We who try are like foreign correspondents" (pp. 256-257).

Robert Hopcke (1989), an American Jungian analyst who has influenced analytical psychology in Britain, states "all sexual orientation is the result of a personal and Archetypal confluence of the masculine, feminine and Androgyny" (p. 187). His approach allows for a non-pathological theory of homosexuality. Hazel Davis (1995) is a Jungian who takes up the issues of prejudice against "homosexuals" and pathologising theories that often lie hidden in the profession. She describes a non-pathological homosexuality using concepts from Friedman, Stoller and Jung. She points out that the concept of the anima/animus allows for masculine or feminine images that are "spontaneously activated to be independent of the gender of the individual" (p. 322) and this understanding of "a dual unconscious gender potential frees the analyst and patient from making gender assumptions" (p. 324). Homosexuality is seen as being compatible with the goals of individuation, which are "the value of wholeness, internal harmony, a steady and reliable self image, the possession of a non-defensive attitude and the capacity to develop intimate relationships being the key issues" (p. 327). The paper calls for equal valuing of what the author calls gay and straight "lifestyles." The Jungian Society of Analytical Psychology has admitted gay candidates to training for many years and has a number of outgay members.

OTHER MENTAL HEALTH PROFESSIONS

The main emphasis in this paper has been on psychoanalytical theory and practitioners. Nevertheless, mental health attitudes toward homosexuality outside the psychoanalytic community changed much earlier. In 1984, the European parliament rejected classifying homosexuality as a mental illness. The Royal College of Psychiatrists supported the equalisation of the age of consent in the same year and it also has a gay and lesbian mental health interest group consisting of 120 members (Nakajima, 2003). In 1986, The Greater London Council, that is the Government of London, called for an end to drug, shock and behaviour therapy to "cure" lesbianism. In 1993, the National Government removed homosexuality from its central computer list of psychiatric disorders.

However, it is important to note the influence of psychoanalytic thought on other health professions in the UK. Psychiatry, as practised in the UK, is eclectic. Some psychiatrists are trained in psychoanalysis while others train in behavioural and pharmacological modalities. Until the 1960s, all of these theoretical approaches shared a common view of homosexuality as pathology. "Despite disagreement about the origins of homosexuality, both behaviourists and analysts assumed that it required treatment" (King and Bartlett, 1999, p. 108). An interdisciplinary team consisting of psychiatrist, psychiatric social worker and psychologist is an integral part of British psychiatric practice. It is also from these core professions that most candidates for psychoanalytic training are recruited. Many psychiatrists who trained at the BPAS often became consultants in the National Health Service (NHS) and were responsible (until the late 1970s) for the work of all members of the multidisciplinary team.

Clinical psychology in the UK has not been very influenced by psychoanalytic theory and practice if examination of the *Clinical Psychology Journal* published by the British Psychological Society is any indication. An examination of the contents of eleven journals from March 1999 through September 2001 revealed no articles with a psychoanalytic viewpoint. The British Psychological Society has a gay and lesbian section since 2000, which publishes its own journal. The Society's equal opportunity policy includes sexual orientation and applies to "academic, professional training and to users of the service." This policy is enshrined in the Code of Conduct Ethical Principles and Guidelines.

The first social work training in the UK took place at the London School of Economics (LSE). Among its student were Clare Winnicott and Betty Joseph, both of whom were to become important figures in British psychoanalysis. Donald Winnicott taught psychoanalytic concepts on this course for many years. Social workers who trained at the LSE have dominated social work for many years and worked psychodynamically. Unsurprisingly, they viewed homosexuality as an illness and subscribed to the psychoanalytical theories of their time.[13]

In the 1980s, the profession became theoretically eclectic and politically conscious. Social workers became involved with minority groups and many "came out" and campaigned for gay and lesbian rights.[14] The National Association of Social Workers now has an Equal Opportunity Policy as part of their Code of Ethics and Practice. All members are required to uphold the code and make a commitment to it at their annual renewal of membership. Its members have been in the vanguard in supporting the rights of gay and lesbians to be parents, to adopt and to foster children.

NOTES

1. Editor's Note: See Greenberg, J. & Mitchell, S. (1983), *Object Relations in Psychoanalytic Theory*. Cambridge, MA: Harvard University Press, for a review of Fairbairn's place in the history of psychoanalytic theory.

2. The notion of pretence was to be resurrected in 1988 by the Thatcher government when homosexual relationships were described as "pretended" in the "clause 28" bill. This bill, intended to prohibit "the promotion" of homosexuality, was passed in an effort to ban any discussion of homosexuality as normal in the schools.

3. Rosen publicly defended and endorsed clause 28 on television.

4. Editor's Note: This linkage has its roots in Freud's early work. See Freud, S. (1905), Three essays on the theory of sexuality. *Standard Edition*, 7:123-246. London: Hogarth Press, 1953.

5. Later in life, Glasser questioned the ubiquitousness of the "homosexual's" sexualization of aggression and wondered if this hypothesized defence also applied to homosexuals who did not need psychoanalytic help (personal communication with psychoanalyst who heard Glasser speak in 1996).

6. When asked by a gay student about the process of applying for psychoanalytic training, a senior member of the BPAS who was teaching a postgraduate course in London replied "that gays were unacceptable for training as they would be unable, because of their homosexuality, to analyse narcissism." After the student complained, however, another member of the BPAS explained to the student body that what they were told at first was not in keeping with the official policy of the Institute of Psychoanalysis (personal communication with student attending the course). There is a strong indication that another gay student was rejected by another psychoanalytic organisation because of his homosexuality whilst being given a "concocted" explanation by the selection committee, leading the applicant's psychoanalyst to make a complaint. She did not accept the explanations given for rejecting her analysand.

7. One writer did not reply to the request for the paper and another refused, citing as the reason for the refusal the preservation of the confidentiality of the paper's case material.

8. In 1948, Anna Freud said "I know from past experience that it is no good for any kind of course or any kind of institution, to permit people with sexual abnormalities"(quoted in Young-Bruehl, 1998, p. 485). Later in life she changed her mind and is quoted aas saying that "a homosexual could be accepted for psychoanalytic training–uncured–if his or her character were suitable" (Young-Bruehl, 1998, p. 327).

9. The magnitude of change that has taken place in British psychoanalytic attitudes towards homosexuality was illustrated recently at BAP's September 2001 Oxford conference in celebration of its 50th birthday. The theme of the conference was "Change." Members who attended a workshop on homosexuality were informed of BAPs Equal Opportunities Policy of February 19, 2000: "The BAP operates an Equal Opportunities Policy; no distinction or discrimination is made on the basis of any variable including ethnicity, religion, gender or sexual orientation. This applies to students, staff, members and patients."

10. One wonders if the writer's use of a pseudonym indicates the level of fear that psychotherapists experienced at being seen even to be associated in 1991 with homosexuality.

11. Editor's Note: See Frommer, M. S. (1995), Countertransference obscurity in the treatment of homosexual patients. In: *Disorienting Sexualities*, ed. T. Domenici & R. C. Lesser. New York: Routledge, pp. 65-82, for such a report.

12. Samuels, a Jungian training analyst, was one of the main protesters at Socarides' visit and refuted his theories in the national press.

13. On a personal note, my first job as a psychiatric social worker was given to me on the condition that I would not disclose my sexual orientation to any of my clients. This was in 1976. Furthermore, this condition from my future employer was conveyed to me by my analyst. At present, social work is more eclectic and it would be difficult to imagine a social worker who is antihomosexually biased getting employment in any area of the public sector.

14. At this time my senior retired and was replaced by an "out" lesbian.

REFERENCES

Balint, M. (1956), Perversions and genitality. In: *Perversions, Psychodynamics and Therapy*, eds. S. Lorand & M. Balint. London: Gramercy Books, pp. 16-27.

Bartlett, A., King, M., Phillips, P. (2001), Straight Talking: An investigation of the attitudes and practice of psychoanalysts and psychotherapists in relation to gays and lesbians. *Brit. J. Psychiat.*, 179:545-549.

Phillips, P., Bartlett, A. & King, M. (2001), Psychotherapists' approaches to gay and lesbian patients/clients: A qualitative study. *Brit. J. Med. Psychol.*, 74:73-84.

Chasseguet-Smirgel, J. (1985a), *The Ego Ideal*. London: Free Association Books.

Chasseguet-Smirgel, J. (1985b), *Perversions and Creativity*. London: Free Association Books.

Cunningham, R. (1991), When is a pervert not a pervert. *Brit. J. Psychother.*, 8(1): 48-70.

Davis, H. (1995), Homosexuality. In: *Zurich '95: Open Questions in Analytical Psychology: Proceedings of the 13th International Congress for Analytical Psychology*, ed. by M. A. Matcon. Einsiedeln: Daimon Verlag, pp. 320-327.

Drescher, J. (1995), Anti-homosexual bias in training. In: *Disorienting Sexualities*, ed. T. Domenici & R. C. Lesser. New York: Routledge, pp. 227-241.

Ellis, M. L. (1994), Lesbians, gay men and psychoanalytic training. *Free Associations*, 4(4):501-517.

Ellis, M. L. (1997), Challenging Socarides. *Feminism & Psychology*, 7(2):287-289.

Fairbairn, R. (1946), The treatment and rehabilitation of sexual offenders. In: *Psychoanalytic Studies Of the Personality*. New York: Routledge, 1952, pp. 289-296.

Frantz, G. (1995), The Psyche's response to the trauma of Aids. In: *Zurich '95: Open questions in Analytical Psychology: Proceedings of the 13th International Congress for Analytical Psychology*, ed. by M. A. Matcon. Einsiedeln: Daimon Verlag, pp. 256-263.

Freud, A. (1949), Some clinical remarks concerning the treatment of cases of male homosexuality (author abstracts). *Int. J. Psychonal.*, 30:195.

Freud, A. (1952), Studies in passivity. In: *The Writings of Anna Freud*, Volume 4. New York: International Universities Press, 1968, pp. 245-259.

Freud, A. (1954), Problems of technique in adult analysis. In: *The Writings of Anna Freud*, Volume 4. New York: International Universities Press, 1968, pp. 337-406.

Freud, S. (1911), Psycho-analytic notes on an autobiographical account of a case of paranoia. *Standard Edition*, 12:1-82. London: Hogarth Press, 1958.

Freud, S. & Rank, O. (1921), Circular Letter. *Body Politic*. Toronto, May 1977, p. 9.

Gillespie, W. (1964), *Life, Sex and Death: Selected Writings*. London: New Library of Psychoanalysis, 1995, pp. 119-129.

Glasser, M. (1977), Homosexuality in adolescence. *Brit. J. Med. Psychol.*, 50:217-225.

Glasser, M. (1979), Some aspects of the role of aggression in sexual perversions. In: *Sexual Deviation*, ed. I. Rosen. Oxford: Oxford University Press, pp. 278-305.

Glover, E. (1939), *Psychoanalysis: A Handbook for Medical Practitioners and Students of Comparative Psychology*. London and New York: Staples Press.

Glover, E. (1960), The problem of male homosexuality. In: *The Roots of Crime: Selected Papers in Psychoanalysis*. New York: International Universities Press, pp. 197-243.

Hopcke, R. (1989), *Jung, Jungians & Homosexuality*. Boston, MA: Shambhala.

Hildebrand, P. (1992), A patient dying with AIDS. *Int. Rev. Psycho-Anal.*, 19:457-69.

Isay, R. (1996), *Becoming Gay: The Journey to Self-Acceptance*. New York: Pantheon.

Izzard, S. (1999), Oedipus–baby and bath water. *Brit. J. Psychother.*, 17(4):44-55.

Jones, D. (2001), Shame, disgust anger and revenge. *Brit. J. Psychother.*, 17(4): 493-503.

King, M. & Bartlett, A. (1999), British psychiatry and homosexuality. *Brit. J. Psychiat.*, 175:106-113.

Klein, M. (1932), *The Psychoanalysis of Children*. London: Hogarth Press.

Kogbara, D. (1995), So ambiguous, this demonised doctor: The Sunday Times Interview. *The Sunday Times* (*News Review*), April 30, p. 8.

Lewes, K. (1988), *The Psychoanalytic Theory of Male Homosexuality*. New York: Simon and Schuster. Reissued as *Psychoanalysis and Male Homosexuality* (1995), Northvale, NJ: Aronson.

Limentani, A. (1979), Clinical types of homosexuality. In: *Sexual Deviation*, ed. I. Rosen. Oxford: Oxford University Press. pp. 195-205.

Mendoza, S. (1997), Criteria of selection of homosexual candidates. *Brit. J. Psychother.*, 13(3):384-394.

Mendoza, S. (2001), Genital and phallic homosexuality. In: *Sexuality: Psychoanalytic Perspectives*, ed. C. Harding. New York/London: Brunner-Routledge, pp. 153-169.

Nakajima, G. A. (2003), The emergence of an international lesbian, gay, and bisexual psychiatric movement. *J. Gay & Lesb. Psychother.*, 7(1/2):165-188.

O'Connor, N. & Ryan, J. (1993), *Wild Desires and Mistaken Identities: Lesbianism & Psychoanalysis*. New York: Columbia University.

Rayner, E. (1990), *Human Development*. London: Routledge.

Rosenfeld, H. (1949), Remarks on the relationship of male homosexuality to paranoia, paranoid anxiety and narcissm. *Int. J. Psycho-Anal.*, 30:36-47.

Rosen, I. (1979), *Sexual Deviation*. Oxford: Oxford University Press.

Samuels, A. (1985), *Jung and the Post-Jungians*. London: Routledge and Kegan Paul.

Segal, H. (1990), Interview with Professor Jacqueline Rose. In: *Women: A Cultural Review*. Oxford: Oxford University Press, pp. 198-214.

Shelley, C. (1998), *Contemporary Perspectives on Psychotherapy and Homosexualities*. London: Free Association Books.

Stoller, R. (1989), *Observing The Erotic Imagination*. New Haven: Yale University Press.

Webb, P. (1994), Bias on the therapist's couch. *Independent*, August 21.

Young-Bruehl, E. (1988), *Anna Freud: A Biography*. New York: Summit.

Zachary, A (2001), Uneasy triangles: A brief overview of the history of homosexuality. *Brit. J. Psychother.*, 17(4):489-492.

From Perversion to Sexual Identity:
Concepts of Homosexuality
and Its Treatment in Germany

Falk Stakelbeck, MD
Udo Frank, MD

SUMMARY. The article describes the attitudes towards gays and lesbians as found in the theory and practice of psychiatry and psychotherapy in Germany. After providing a brief historical background, it presents the concepts of homosexuality prevailing in psychiatry, psychoanalysis and sexology after 1945, primarily focusing on West Germany. In the early years of West Germany, the ideas of anthropological psychiatry, psychoanalysis and those fields of sexology dealing with this subject exclusively followed normative concepts. During the subsequent period of social liberalization this normative fixation was revised by a new generation of sexologists. During this period, Fritz Morgenthaler also formulated

Falk Stakelbeck, psychiatrist and psychotherapist, trained for his specialisation in Switzerland and Germany. He is Psychotherapist in a hospital in Munich and is in analytic training at the Akademie für Psychoanalyse, Munich. He is Co-Chairman of the German Association of Gays in the Health Service (Bundesarbeitsgemeinschaft Schwule im Gesundheitswesen, BASG e.V.).

Udo Frank is Psychiatrist, Neurologist and Psychotherapist (DGPPN) and is Medical Vice-Director of a forensic department at a psychiatric hospital in Ravensburg, South-Germany. He is Co-Chairman of the German Association of Gays in the Health Service (Bundesarbeitsgemeinschaft Schwule im Gesundheitswesen, BASG e.V.).

The authors would like to thank the members of the *Bundesarbeitsgemeinschaft Schwule im Gesundheitswesen (BASG e.V.)* for allowing them to discuss this article at their meeting and for providing financial support for its translation.

[Haworth co-indexing entry note]: "From Perversion to Sexual Identity: Concepts of Homosexuality and Its Treatment in Germany." Stakelbeck, Falk, and Udo Frank. Co-published simultaneously in *Journal of Gay & Lesbian Psychotherapy* (The Haworth Medical Press, an imprint of The Haworth Press, Inc.) Vol. 7, No. 1/2, 2003, pp. 23-46; and: *The Mental Health Professions and Homosexuality: International Perspectives* (ed: Vittorio Lingiardi, and Jack Drescher) The Haworth Medical Press, an imprint of The Haworth Press, Inc., 2003, pp. 23-46. Single or multiple copies of this article are available for a fee from The Haworth Document Delivery Service [1-800-HAWORTH, 9:00 a.m. - 5:00 p.m. (EST). E-mail address: getinfo@haworthpressinc.com].

10.1300/J236v07n01_03

the first psychoanalytical conception of a non-pathological homosexuality in Germany. The psychoanalytic concepts of the last few years emphasize the different modi of sexual identity. After homosexuality ceased to be a diagnosis in itself, it became impossible to determine a consistent psychiatric model. There are few empirical studies documenting the actual situation of gay and lesbian patients or of gay and lesbian health care professionals in the German health service. Consequently, what is known about their current situation is based primarily on anecdotal evidence and indirect references. This article is the first to report on three surveys about the admission policies of German psychoanalytic institutes toward gay and lesbian applicants and candidates, including previously unpublished data showing changes in institute policies. Attitudes in the mental health fields mirror the general social climate and range from pathologization and other more subtle forms of homophobia to almost complete acceptance. *[Article copies available for a fee from The Haworth Document Delivery Service: 1-800-HAWORTH. E-mail address: <getinfo@haworthpressinc. com> Website: <http://www.HaworthPress.com> © 2003 by The Haworth Press, Inc. All rights reserved.]*

KEYWORDS. Developmental theory, gay/lesbian mental health professionals, gay/lesbian patients, German Association of Gays in the Health Service (BASG e.V.), German psychiatry, German psychoanalysis, homosexuality, mental health, psychoanalytic training, sexology

HISTORICAL BACKGROUND

In Germany, as in almost all western industrialized nations, the integration of gays and lesbians into society has increased over the last three decades. Changes in the laws on homosexuality are a good example of this process of integration. Until the beginning of the 1990s, the penal code of the old West Germany remained in force[1] as an expression of the still-existing will to penalize homosexuality. However, the relatively recent introduction of a civil law on gay and lesbian partnerships now grants unprecedented legal protection to gay people for the first time in Germany. This new partnership law does not afford same-sex relationships the same rights as heterosexual relationships, but a gay or lesbian relationship is being recognized as a legally protected right.

These protections can be contrasted with the preceding decade. Until the beginning of the 1990s, gay men were subject to criminal prosecution and female homosexuality did not even exist in the eyes of the law. The instrument of gay men's persecution was article (or paragraph) 175 of the criminal code. First drafted after the German Reich was founded under Bismarck in 1871, article 175 eventually became the law in all German states. From a legal, historical perspective, this represented a step backwards; in many European countries, including some of the smaller German states, homosexuality had not been penalized for decades after the adoption of the Napoleonic code.

The *Wissenschaftlich-humanitäre Komitee* [Scientific Humanitarian Committee] (WhK) in Berlin, founded in 1897, was the first political organization to demand equal civil rights for homosexuals.[2] The acknowledged political aim of the WhK was the abolition of paragraph 175. The founding of the WhK also marked the birth of the first gay liberation movement in the world. The theories of its founder, the sexologist Magnus Hirschfeld, were closely linked to the political aims of the movement. His idea of a "third sex,"[3] which assigns homosexuals to a kind of psychosexual hermaphroditic position between the sexes, was also an attempt at political emancipation beyond this daring speculation. His argument that homosexuality was a natural state was intended to convince legislators that the criminal prosecution of male homosexuality was a futile endeavor.

However, in the end, the efforts of the WhK did not lead to the abolition of article 175. After the Nazis rose to power, in 1935 they made the article even more restrictive. In its harsher version, article 175 made homosexual "intentions," without the necessity of any accompanying homosexual act, a punishable offense. Many "homosexuals" were later sent to concentration camps and exterminated.[4] The theories informing that policy grew out of two lines of thought. On the one hand, researchers were looking for a biological origin–and therefore for a possible treatment or cure–for homosexuality. On the other hand, the distinction between homosexual and heterosexual "identities" was abandoned. Homosexual acts were regarded in isolation without reference to the overall personality. Because health was fundamentally considered to be a matter of population policy during the Third Reich, homosexual behavior posed a threat to the health and reproduction of the entire population and had to be persecuted at all costs.

In West Germany after the war, article 175 remained in force unchanged. Homosexuals who had survived the concentration camps continued to be subject to criminal prosecution in the early years of West Germany. Under these conditions, it was impossible to continue the traditions of the first gay liberation movement. Psychiatric and psychoanalytic theories of that period–and the extent of homosexual pathology that they proclaimed–further increased the pressure on homosexuals.

After the criminal law was liberalized in 1969 and 1973, a gay liberation movement quickly formed in the wake of the student and women's movements. In the early days of the gay liberation movement, its prominent representatives formulated a theory of homosexuality which predominantly took the form of social criticism. Picking up the argument that homosexuality was a force that endangered social structures–a central theme of previous theories–these new formulations reinterpreted this as a positive function. However, social theories initially had no effect on the theories of psychiatry and psychoanalysis. After the 1970s, the gay liberation movement was critically assessed by a new generation of sexologists who published empirical studies and questioned the ideological entanglements of the traditional theories of psychiatry and psychoanalysis.

Until the beginning of the 1980s, psychoanalysis followed the literature of the French, British and American schools. The theories of pathology that were presented in these articles apparently met with a good response. In 1984, Fritz Morgenthaler published the first theory–in the German-speaking countries–of a non-pathological genesis of homosexuality. From about the mid-eighties, the theories of traditional psychoanalysis were questioned by feminist psychoanalysis and the ideas about treatment methods. Both of these forces led to a change in the formulation of theories on gays and lesbians.

THE EARLY YEARS OF WEST GERMANY

The Penal Code

After the Second World War, the restrictive version of paragraph 175, which had been tightened by the Nazis, remained in force for several more decades. However, in 1969, homosexual acts between adult men ceased to be a criminal offense. Nevertheless, a higher age of consent for gay men (21) than the age of consent for heterosexuals (16) remained in force.[5] In 1973, the age of homosexual consent was lowered from 21 to 18 while the heterosexual age of consent remained the same.[6]

Psychiatry and Sexology

In the early years of West Germany, psychiatrists and sexologists both exclusively discussed concepts which maintained that homosexuality was psychopathological. This represented a movement of these disciplines away from the positions of both Magnus Hirschfeld and Freud. It was argued in this era that the extent of "homosexual pathology" always corresponded to a serious personality disorder; homosexuals were described as having problems with structural level, development of the super-ego, affect differentiation, object and self-perception, etc.

Although one might suppose that a theory of a biological disposition toward homosexuality would certainly resonate with the underlying premises of sexology and psychiatry–as opposed to the theories of psychoanalysis–biological theories regarding homosexuality's etiology were rarely formulated during this period. The representatives of anthropological psychiatry, whose most eminent proponents included V. E. von Gebsattel (1929, 1932, 1950), H. Kunz (1942, 1954), O. Schwarz (1932), and O. Strauß (1930), gained great influence in the formulation of the term "perversion" in orthodox medicine; the term always referred to homosexuality (Giese, 1967; Dannecker, 1978). These theories were supported by the sociologists A. Gehlen (1940) and H. Schelsky (1955) as well. According to these authors, the biological drive for reproduction is manifest not only in human sexuality, but also in the (implicit) aim of promoting and supporting social institutions, and in this case particularly the institution of marriage. They regarded all forms of sexuality that deviated from the reproductive drive and from conservative institutional support as perversions, rather than a normal variant of human sexuality. In other words, "perversion"–that is the practice of nonheterosexual, genital intercourse–was regarded as an attack on social institutions. It was further argued that perverse behavior is destructive because it could become subject of a progression, an "addictive cycle" (v. Gebsattel, 1932).

The anthropological psychiatry outlined here forms the theoretical frame of reference for the sexologist H. Giese, who was well-known beyond the world of science and instrumental in initiating the liberalization of the criminal law during this period of political restoration in West Germany. The central theme of Giese's *Der homosexuelle Mann in der Welt* [The Homosexual Man in the World] (1964) was the desire to provide homosexuals with a permanent place in society, or, at least in theory, a place within the moral order. Giese's theoretical strategy was to divide homosexuals into those who are living in a relationship (*gebundene*) and those who are not (*ungebundene*). He regarded homosexual relationships as a possible way of regulating the sexuality of the "homosexual." Those behavioral patterns that might lead to an "addictive cycle" (promiscuity, anonymity, differentiation of the sexual stimuli without sexual satisfaction) were thought to require control. According to Giese, homosexuals in a relationship represented a variation of normal sexuality. Their relationships were not perverse because their sexuality and the "destructiveness" linked to it (that is, the antisocial features) had been defused by the relationship. Unfortunately, in order to advance his normal variant theory of homosexuality, and to downplay the association between unconventional sexual behaviors and psychopathology, Giese had to ignore specific differences between the sexuality of homosexuals and heterosexuals. However, despite all of Giese's theoretical efforts, the mental health majority's opinions regarding homosexuality remained unchanged.

Psychoanalysis

During the Third Reich, the institutional framework of psychoanalysis had been largely destroyed. In the post-war period, psychoanalysis began to re-form itself and tried to catch up with international developments. Expanded models of homosexuality were not formulated in West Germany, but the works of British and American authors, including M. Klein (1932), E. Bergler and L. Eidelberg (1933), G. Bychowski (1961) and C. Socarides (1968) were translated and adopted. Despite their diverse theoretical backgrounds within psychoanalysis, these authors shared a common formulation of homosexuality as a preoedipal complex which formed the basis for later developing adult homosexuality. They held that the frustrating experiences with the primary object or phantasmic fixations (Klein) were the conditions for a persistence of the primary identification with the mother and which then prevented a secondary identification with the parent of the same gender. The persistence of this preoedipal complex—with undifferentiated self and object imagines and unresolved conflicts of separation and aggression—interferes with the formation of adult, heterosexual psychic structures. In theory, this expansion of the presumed psychopathology of homosexuals, which was now said to encompass all aspects of their personality (structural levels, development of the super-ego, affect differentiation, object and self-perception, etc.), was linked to the notion of a preoedipal matrix. This meant that the express aim of treatment inherent in this notion was to change a homosexual's sexual orientation towards a heterosexual choice of object.

BETWEEN LIBERALIZATION AND INTEGRATION

While the post-war years' debate over the liberalization of Germany's criminal law was dominated by socially conservative professional voices, a changed climate would emerge after the student revolts of the 1960s, the women's movement and the early gay liberation movement of the 1970s. Each of these had an influence on the theories of homosexuality that emerged over the following years. The early gay liberation movement, for example, argued primarily on the basis of social theory. The role of the homosexual outsider was now regarded as a positive factor and interpreted as a motivation to change society. The changed social climate and the social movements were critically evaluated by a new generation of sexologists. The history of psychoanalysis was being re-evaluated. The underlying assumptions of fundamental, historical psychoanalytic concepts, such as penis envy or the death instinct, were questioned. Consequently, during this period the first psychoanalytic developmental theory hypothesizing the existence of a non-pathological homosexuality was published in German.

Sexology

The publication of M. Dannecker and R. Reiche's empirical study *Der gewöhnliche Homosexuelle* [The Ordinary Homosexual] (1974) represented an abrupt break with sexological practice of the early years in West Germany. Looking back, their work marks a turning point in the theoretical debate on homosexuality in Germany. Dannecker and Reiche's work was the first empirical study that described an ideal type of "normal" homosexual beyond the limited clinical viewpoint which focused on psychopathology.

The authors interpreted their large pool of data (789 questionnaires completed by homosexual men) in the framework of psychoanalytic theory, but kept their critical distance by also adding a social theoretical perspective. The authors examined socialization in the gay male subculture (behavior in bars, saunas, etc.), coming-out, career and sexual practices. The data showed that a vast majority of homosexual men were living in long-term relationships. In contrast to Giese's earlier assertion, the authors found no significant difference between single gay men and gay men in relationships in regard to having multiple sexual partners. The study also drew attention, for the first time, to the social phenomenon of homophobia as practiced by gay men, which the authors referred to as a "collective neurosis." By this they referred to the observation that gay men themselves expressed critical or unaccepting feelings toward any effeminate aspects of homosexual men.[7]

Dannecker and Reiche's emphasis on the differences between homosexuals and heterosexuals (for example, in the realm of promiscuous behavior or the frequency of anal intercourse) argued against then-prevailing sexological views. However, by arguing for gay men's ability to achieve social conformity, they also challenged the psychoanalytic orthodoxy. Previously, anthropological and early sexological discussions of homosexuality primarily focused on a postulated (hetero)social norm, on which they based their notion of health. In *Der gewöhnliche Homosexuelle*, some of the subjective experiences of gay men were spelled out; it was the first time that the German literature presented concepts like coming out, homosexual self-loathing, etc., in a scientific context.

Dannecker and Reiche also took issue with the gay liberationist position which considered homosexuality to be an expression of the social and sexual *avant-garde*. In their discussion of promiscuity, for example, they argued that neither anthropological psychiatry's critical interpretations, nor the early gay liberation movement's affirmative interpretations of promiscuity were accurate. Promiscuity, they asserted, did not represent an act capable of either changing or destroying the fabric of society. Instead, they interpreted the meaning of the phenomenon (1) on an individual basis as an emotional splitting mechanism between the sexual drive and the striving for tenderness and (2) on a collective basis as a search for new forms of satisfying one's needs.

Psychoanalysis

Concurrent with social liberalization toward homosexuality in Germany, critical positions were also being formulated toward the theoretical foundations of psychoanalytical theories. As in other countries, the historical and methodological assumptions of psychoanalysis were being questioned and challenged. Initially, these theoretical discussions remained on an abstract level and had no direct effect on psychoanalytic treatment approaches and theorizing about homosexuality. Important analytic journals and renowned publishers continued to print articles by other European theorists such as Chasseguet-Smirgel (1975, 1984), McDougall (1978) and Masud R. Khan (1979), who continued to argue for the pathological perspective of a preoedipal homosexual matrix.

The first postwar theory of a non-pathological homosexuality by the Swiss psychoanalyst Fritz Morgenthaler (1984),[8] to the present day remains the most famous paper published in German on this subject.[9] Three "decisive points"– which Morgenthaler explicitly considers to be distinct from the phases of the classical libidinal development–play a most important role in his theory of a normative homosexual development. In Morgenthaler's opinion, these decisive points do not represent points of fixation but of "progressive dispositions."

In a first stage in early childhood, the prehomosexual child initially reacts to the unavoidable disruptions in the construction of the self-image during the separation and rapprochement phase (Mahler, Pine and Bergman, 1975) with an over-cathexis of autoerotic activities. This over-cathexis of autoerotic activities is the result of an accelerated development of the sexual drive. In contrast, the development of the ego is relatively retarded when compared to heterosexuals. According to Morgenthaler, the fact that the development of the sexual drive and of the ego no longer occur at the same time is not a pathological phenomenon, but a possible reaction to the conflicts in the separation phase.[10] Because of the relatively retarded development of the ego the control over aggressive and sexual impulses is weakened.

In order to guarantee a balanced development of the self-image, autoerotic activities become very important, or–in the language of drive psychology–over-cathected. Autoerotic activities also play an important role in the further development in order to regulate self-esteem. Autoerotic activities, which are so closely tied to physical experiences, are, however, transformed in further development. For areas that are in a greater distance from physical experience, Morgenthaler assumes that the autoerotic experience is transformed into the "over-cathexis" of the autonomy in the self-image. The autonomy in the self-image takes the part of the earlier sexual activity. In the sexual organization this is represented by an interest in persons of the same sex.

The prehomosexual child then enters the oedipal phase with a disposition to desire objects of the same sex. The parents react to this interest initially with the socially expected role patterns. In correlation with parental expectations, role patterns, etc., the desire of the prehomosexual child is now initially directed towards the parent of the opposite sex. The child receives strong feelings of rejection from the parent of the same sex, to which it in turn reacts with a strong castration threat anxiety. At the height of the oedipal conflict, the sexual characteristics of the parent of the same sex are discovered. The rival, to whom the prehomosexual child wanted to submit out of fear, becomes an object of sexual interest. The relationship to the parent of the same sex therefore has two aspects: passive submission and narcissistic conquest. According to Morgenthaler, both modi are an integral part of every homosexual relationship. During the third decisive point during puberty, the integration of the adolescent's own wishes and social assumptions about homosexuality become important.[11]

MOMENTS OF INTEGRATION

At the end of the 1980s, the appearance of AIDS significantly changed German society's attitudes towards gay men. The setback to civil rights that was initially expected did not occur. For many people, gay men became visible for the first time. Safer sex campaigns spoke very openly about gay sex. The creation of German AIDS organizations earned gay activists increased respect. Sympathy with the victims of the disease was probably another factor in increasing tolerance and acceptance. It is one of the paradoxes of AIDS that its appearance propelled the social integration of gay people. In 1994, paragraph 175 was repealed from the criminal code. Soon afterwards, the first debates about creating legal forms of same-sex partnerships began.

Psychiatry

In 1992, the World Health Organization's tenth revision of the International Classification of Diseases (ICD-10) closely followed the American scheme of the Diagnostic and Statistical Manual (DSM). Like the DSM, the ICD-10 excluded homosexuality as a diagnosis in psychiatric medicine. Insofar as the ICD-10 was adopted *in toto*, there was no debate in Germany about individual diagnoses. In contrast to the United States–where the question of the pathology of homosexuality was subject to intense medical and psychiatric controversy (Bayer, 1981)–the positions of the American-dominated, international psychiatric-medical discussion became binding for West German psychiatry without any parallel discussion taking place.

At the same time, the remaining influence of the classical German psychiatric schools (e.g., E. Bleuler, K. Jaspers, K. Schneider, the anthropological school, etc.) continued to diminish in favor of a socio-psychiatric perspective. The relationship between academic psychiatry and psychoanalysis in Germany could best be described as one of critical distance. For instance, psychoanalysis did not enter the academic world via psychiatry, but via internal medicine. For a variety of reasons, an integration model of the psyche, in the form offered by psychoanalysis, was not established in psychiatry in Germany. Some fields of research now favor biological theories more strongly. Thus, there is no discernible unified model of homosexuality in psychiatry and the textbooks of the last two decades therefore contain different positions. Many have simply deleted earlier chapters on homosexuality (Berger, 1999; Tölle, 1999). Others contain practical advice on the therapeutic position and different aspects of specifically gay or lesbian conflicts (Möller, 1995; Dörner and Plog, 1996). Some others still list theories on the strong pathology of homosexuality (Frank, 1993).[12]

Psychoanalysis

The most common reference point for depatholigization shared by many analysts can be found in Otto Kernberg's theories (1997). The observation that gay people differ from one another and–speaking from a clinical viewpoint–function at different structural levels of personality, is a perspective which is increasingly being accepted by many analysts. The question of how homosexuality is to be assessed on a higher, that is, neurotic structural level remains. According to Kernberg's earlier work, homosexual men can achieve the ability of comprehensive object relationships at this level. However, they do not identify with their fathers during the oedipal period. Therefore, they have no comprehensive, that is, sexual relationships with adult women and therefore do not truly accept the function of fatherhood. Because of this lack of identification with the heterosexual father, they are said to be compulsively tied to homosexual relationships.[13]

Classical psychoanalysts attempted to develop a developmental theory which was to be as coherent as possible and able to claim universal validity. However, feminist and relational psychoanalysts have criticized universalizing development models and these criticisms form the theoretical background for discussions regarding non-pathological homosexual development. Feminist psychoanalysts have shown that universality has, at least to date, always been tied to a male reference model (Benjamin, 1988). From this perspective, all of psychoanalysis' developmental claims, such as the outcome of the

Oedipus complex, could be critically re-evaluated. In addition to the feminist critique of psychoanalysis, the epistemological assumptions of psychoanalysis' universalizing tendencies were also being questioned in regard to the practice and theory of treatment. In treatment methodology, a model that places more emphasis on the actual relationship between therapist and patient, or the actual transference and countertransference, than on the reconstruction of the past was gaining wider acceptance (Mitchell and Aron, 1999). In the "meanings discovered" model of treatment, it is argued that meanings grow out of a therapeutic relationship and that they are not necessarily "discovered" by observation of repetitions from the patient's childhood.

In the early 1990s, the gay-affirmative psychoanalytic work of Americans R. Isay (1990) and R. Friedman (1993) were translated into German. In addition, B. Gissrau (1993), E. S. Poluda-Korte (1993) and S. Castendyk (1998) published in Germany theories on lesbian development. Then, in 2000,[14] R. Reiche, one of the authors of *Der gewöhnliche Homosexuelle* [The Ordinary Homosexual]–and by then one of the most prolific German psychoanalysts–presented his views on an "ordinary path in the development of homosexuality." In addition, a number of case studies were published in the 90s whose tenor showed noticeable changes (Henningsen, 1995; Junkert-Tress and Reister, 1995; Le Soldat, 2000; Reiche, 2000). In contrast to Morgenthaler's approach of describing general aspects in development of the self, the approach of these later authors was to place their emphasis on the development of sexual identity.

Isay's *Being Homosexual* (1989) was translated into German a year after it had first been published in America.[15] His vivid descriptions of the erotic bond between the prehomosexual child and his father also left a mark outside the analytical field. The erotically desired father, as opposed to psychoanalysis' historically absent father, now appears regularly in every possible and sometimes surprising context, even coming-out brochures. References to Isay's work also appear in the clinical literature in discussions of non-pathological homosexuality, although not in substantive discussions. The citation usually does not go beyond a mere reference. One exception is M. Dannecker (2000), who took up Isay's theories of secondary effeminization as an expression of oedipal desires directed towards the father. Following Isay, Dannecker introduced the concept of a "femininity push." This referred to the absence of gender conformity, as this phenomena is known in the social sciences.

The publication of the German translation of R. Friedman's *Male Homosexuality* (1993) depicted gay men for the first time as having differing structural levels of personality organization. Freidman's work reflected not only an interest in depathologizing homosexuality, but also the increasing level of importance being given in German psychoanalysis to a concept developed by American researchers–that of "gender identity." The concepts of core gender identity, gender role identity and sexual orientation form the background of his theories. Friedman theorized that homosexuality grows out of a disturbed or partially disturbed gender identity of the prehomosexual boy (effeminacy, unmanliness). a position which received some critical reviews (Dannecker, 1990; Künzler, 1991).[16] In comparison to other normalizing theories of homosexuality, the concept of core gender identity offers the advantage that an undisturbed one makes the argument for a development that is essentially not pathological in its "core." In other words, gays and lesbians may be different from heterosexuals, but essentially their gender identity is not disturbed–although it is possible to assimilate later experiences in a way that may lead to conflict and hence to a disturbed gender role identity.[17]

Friedman explicitly presents his theories in the context of a biological, psychosocial theoretical approach. The German authors briefly discussed below attempt to formulate their theories of development from a purely psychodynamic approach that primarily refers to interaction and identification processes during early childhood or the analytical process. Reiche (2000), for example, argues that everyone has always been either heterosexual or homosexual. The choice of a partner of the same sex is an autonomous element in the psychological organization of the gay individual, and not a symptom, Therefore, long-term analysis can only determine a certain point retrospectively at which someone attributes the term "homosexual" to a certain memory. According to Reiche, an analysis cannot go beyond a point of "before" as is described in some psychoanalytical case studies. A gay man or a lesbian woman will come to a point in their memory at which they perceive themselves as "different," and this "difference" is later interpreted as homosexuality. Because clinical experience cannot determine, but merely postulates a "before" ("biological constitution," "genes," "pre-natal hormone levels," "preoedipal core complex," "partially disturbed gender identity during childhood," etc.), Reiche proposes the following idea: Both gender identity and the choice of an object of the same sex are established simultaneously as one process. He suggests this happens before the child reaches the age of four. Although Reiche does not specify the details of this process, the primary objects are thought to play an important role. For the parents, a little boy is not just a little boy; he also has a certain meaning for them. They convey this meaning via messages that are read and misread by the prehomosexual child, although Reiche does not believe that parents send out a subconscious message to their child encouraging him or her to become homosexual.[18]

In the 1990s, models of a non-pathological female homosexuality were introduced in Germany for the first time. These ideas were preceded by revised views on male homosexuality; more importantly, they were preceded by the revision of female identity development put forth by feminist psychoanalysts. This approach questioned the use of a heterosexual male frame of reference as a standard of normative development. Psychoanalysts who describe the development of a non-pathological female homosexuality differentiate their model from the male frame of reference and from the developmental model of female heterosexuality as well. For example, B. Gissrau (1993) and E. S. Poluda-Korte (1993) showed how female heterosexuality forms the frame of reference in the developmental models of the English and French schools. In their own work, they reinterpret the dynamic formulations of heterosexual female predecessors, as in the example of the girl child longing for the mother's body. Gissrau (1993), for example, suspects that in the early years, the relationship between a mother and a prehomosexual daughter has more intensive erotic undertones when compared to the relationship between a mother and a pre-heterosexual daughter. The mother responds to the erotic desire of the daughter with acceptance rather than punishment. The prehomosexual daughter consequently forms an "erotic object representation" early in life which compensates for all forms of narcissistic offense. This object representation becomes the basis for the further stages of development in the oedipal phase and puberty. During the Oedipal years, Gissrau interprets any gender-atypical or tomboyish behavior of a prehomosexual girl as a reaction to the mother's presumed desires for a male partner; the prehomosexual daughter adapts her behavior to satisfy these presumed desires.

Poluda-Korte (1993) also makes the early desire of the daughter the centerpiece of her theories. She claims that all daughters, including pre-heterosexual women, see their mothers as a lover during the first years of their life. The interaction with the parents, however, conveys a homosexual taboo at a very early stage. Every daughter therefore experiences not only the exclusion from the parental sexual relation during the early separation and individuation phase (Mahler, Pine and Bergman, 1975), but also has to overcome the homosexual taboo. Most women respond to this taboo by identifying with the mother and her female functions ("motherhood"). Prehomosexual women, however, respond to this taboo differently; they identify with the mother to a lesser extent and settle upon her as their object choice instead. Poluda-Korte further hypothesizes that the reason for this different path can be found in the parents' greater tolerance of their daughter's homosexual desires.

In contrast to the theories mentioned to far, S. Castendyk (1998) introduced another dynamic theory in which the homosexual choice of object is the result of unconscious oedipal conflicts. Homosexuality is considered exclusively to result from oedipal conflicts that revolve around the issues of lust, rivalry, etc. In addition to the previously discussed elements of sexual organization–core gender identity, gender role identity and choice of sexual object–"sexual positioning" plays a decisive role in Castendyk's theory. The term refers to gender-specific behavior during erotic dialogue, flirting and sexual encounters. Freud (1920) refers to erotic positioning as a sexual attitude and characterizes it as either passive or active. According to Castendyk, sexual positioning is established during the relatively late oedipal stage of development. Echoing I. Fast (1984), she claims that establishment of one's gender identity requires overcoming envy of the other gender. This also requires abandoning omnipotent fantasies of being both sexes at once. Castendyk's central hypothesis is that in a further stage of development, the omnipotent fantasy of belonging to both sexes has to be abandoned in order to realize erotic desire. The desire for the other becomes possible only by "limiting" oneself to one position in the erotic game; the establishment of one sexual position requires the relinquishment of the other. In a further stage, the choice of sexual object on the basis of sexual positioning is established. This positioning may very well be the result of conflict-ridden conditions. For example, a child with a frigid mother may not be able to satisfy its lust by identifying with the parent of the same sex and may "prefer" to identify with the sexual position of the parent of the other sex.

The appearance of psychodynamic development models of a non-pathological homosexuality marks a changed climate in Germany. Of course, a theoretical overview does not say whether these theories have been acknowledged and accepted by the majority of practicing psychoanalysts. However, psychoanalytic theories that perpetuate the notion of homosexuality per se as pathological have not been published for some years. It is also worth noting that some of the contributions of the above-mentioned theoreticians were presented in mainstream psychoanalytic venues. Reiche presented his theories at the fiftieth anniversary of the *Deutsche Psychoanalytische Vereinigung* (DPV) [German Psychoanalytical Association]. Podula-Korte published several articles on the "lesbian complex" in *Psyche*, the most renowned German psychoanalytical journal, and Friedman's translated book was published as part of a highly respected scientific series.

THE EXPERIENCE OF GAY AND LESBIAN PATIENTS/CLIENTS

What is known about the actual experience of gays and lesbians who are seeking psychiatric or psychotherapeutic treatment in Germany? Surprisingly, there is hardly any literature and virtually no empirical studies on the subject. The German professional literature, however, is now beginning to deal with the specific aspects of psychotherapeutic treatment of gays and lesbians (Rauchfleisch, 2001; Symalla and Walther, 1997), indicating that the situation for those seeking help has improved. There is also an increasing self-help literature for gay people (Siems, 1980; Köllner, 1994). The current situation can, however, be mostly understood on the basis of anecdotal evidence and indirect references.

We are not aware of any recent individual cases, published in professional literature or documented elsewhere, in which patients received openly homophobic treatment from their therapists. Surveys among psychotherapists (Wiesendanger, 2001) and case studies published by therapists show that there is a surprising amount of reflection and no prejudice in the treatment of gay and lesbian patients (e.g., Henningsen, 1995; Junkert-Tress and Reister, 1995; Le Soldat, 2000; Reiche, 2000), irrespective of the therapist's own sexual orientation.

On the other hand many gay and lesbian clients deliberately look for gay or lesbian therapists (Heinrich and Biechele, 1997). Their motives for doing so may be fear of open or covert homophobia during their therapy or at least of a continuation of the heterosexism they experience in everyday life. They also hope to come across more empathy with regard to certain subjects or some knowledge about gay and lesbian (sub)culture. For these reasons among others, some gay communities in larger cities have developed specialized psychological and psychotherapeutic advice centers. These include the *Schwulenberatung Berlin* [Gay Advice Center Berlin] or the *Psychologische Lesben- und Schwulenberatung Rhein-Neckar PLUS* [Psychological Lesbian and Gay Advice Centre Rhine-Neckar Region] in Mannheim. These centers are partially financed by public funds and offer differentiated advice and treatment by and for gays and lesbians. They offer guidance for individuals and couples, therapy-assisted coming-out, courses on introspection and assertiveness, contact seminars, services for gay and lesbian psychiatric patients and drug addicts, and weekend seminars on the subject of gay parenting.

The financial policies of health insurance companies offer further anecdotal evidence on attitudes toward gay and lesbian patients. Outpatient psychotherapeutic treatment is generally paid for by statutory health insurance, which is used by the vast majority of people. Before treatment can begin, however, the therapist has to send a report, which does not include the patient's name, to an expert who checks the medical indication and decides whether to pay for treatment. In a workshop of the *Verband lesbischer Psychologinnen und schwuler Psychologen in Deutschland e.V.* (VLSP) [Association of Lesbian and Gay Psychologists in Germany] on the subject (Doll, 2001), the attending therapists said that reports which openly referred to the patient's homosexuality had never been rejected. The impression was that most health insurance experts did not seem to regard homosexuality as "pathological," nor does it have to be psychodynamically discussed in the reports. Nonetheless, the therapists writing the reports felt unsure as to how to write about their clients' homosexuality without risking that the insurance companies reject paying for the treatment.

THE EXPERIENCE OF GAY AND LESBIAN PROFESSIONALS

What is the situation of openly gay or lesbian mental health workers in the areas of psychiatry, psychotherapy and psychoanalysis? This question can also be answered indirectly on the basis of anecdotal evidence. We will describe the current situation by looking at the experiences of openly gay or lesbian candidates applying for psychotherapy training, the opportunities for scientific research into gay and lesbian subjects, and also the existence and the topics of gay and lesbian groups in the health service or psychology and psychotherapy.

The Situation of Openly Gay and Lesbian Trainees

In Germany, as mentioned above, psychotherapy is paid for by all compulsory statutory and private health insurance companies. Apart from an appropriate diagnosis, the health insurance companies also require that the therapist be trained in a method recognized by them. These methods include behavioral therapy and psychoanalysis–or their modified methods, such as analytically oriented psychotherapy, group therapy, etc.[19]

Training is open to psychologists and medical practitioners. Apart from these formal criteria, candidates also have to prove their personal suitability during selective interviews. Behavioral psychology, unlike psychoanalysis, does not use developmental psychology to pathologize homosexuality. We can only assume that the overall situation for potential trainees is quite favorable in this area. However, we were unable to ascertain whether candidates are asked at all about their sexual orientation during the initial interview. There are no known cases of openly gay candidates being rejected for courses in behavioral therapy in recent years and some teachers at the institutes were openly gay. Some candidates, however, have complained that the study of sexuality in general, and of homosexuality in particular, is rarely included in their training–even when such training would be necessary (Rimmler, 1998). The fear of having to deal with prejudices when coming out, the lack of openly gay and lesbian role models among the teachers, and insults because of irrational interpretation of their sexual orientation by colleagues are, however, facets of the subjective experiences of gay and lesbian candidates (Rimmler, 1998).

Although the issue of excluding gay and lesbian candidates from training in behavioral psychology has not been the subject of empirical study, the rejection of gay and lesbian candidates for training in psychoanalysis has been examined in relevant studies. In the early 1980s, several men from the *Bundesarbeitsgemeinschaft Schwule im Gesundheitswesen* (BASG) [German Association of Gays in the Health Service] had their applications for training in psychoanalysis rejected after they were interviewed. In a survey of 26 psychoanalytic training institutes in West Germany, only 14 responded to the questionnaire. Of these 14 institutes, not one explicitly stated that gay and lesbian candidates were rejected. Their replies were, however, formal and could also be read as "In principle we don't, but . . ." (BASG, 1985). These formal replies, however, contradicted the experiences of candidates to whom it was made clear after their first interview that they would not be admitted. In another survey of 41 institutes in Germany, Switzerland and Austria in 1991/92, 34 of them responded. Five institutes stated, for the first time, that they admitted homosexual candidates. Two institutes criticized previous admission policies and a further six reported internal discussions about admission policies (Rauchfleisch, 1993). In a second survey carried out by BASG in 1993/94, 46 institutes replied: 7 German, 2 Swiss and 2 Austrian institutes unambiguously stated that they admitted homosexual candidates. Another 10 institutes in Germany, one in Switzerland and one in Austria confirmed that they trained homosexual candidates or employed homosexual teachers. There were still a number of institutes that supplied formal replies which gave no indication of their actual policies.[20]

The surveys were not meant to be representative studies, but rather an "inventory" of the then-current policies regarding the situation of gay and lesbian candidates. Although the true policies of many institutes could not be established, the few definite statements show a distinct change during the period from 1984 to the beginning of the 1990s. Openly homosexual candidates were admitted for the first time during this period. Meanwhile gays and lesbians are able to qualify in psychoanalysis in Germany. Because the attitudes of the institutes vary greatly, candidates may be required to move to a different area. The trainees who we are personally acquainted with are all attending institutes of the *Deutsche Psychoanalytische Gesellschaft* (DPG) [German Psychoanalytical Society], the *Deutsche Gesellschaft für Analytische Psychologie* (DGAP) [German Society for Analytical Psychology] or independent institutes. Not one trainee at the *Deutsche Psychoanalytische Vereinigung* (DPV) [German Psychoanalytical Association], the only association that is a member of the International Psychoanalytical Association (IPA), is known to us. In the early 1980s, an openly gay candidate was initially admitted to a course in Gießen by the local course committee of a DPV institute. The case was then referred to the national, and possibly also to an international committee; the candidate was subsequently rejected (BASG, 1984; Künzler, 1992). We do not know whether the DPV institutes have changed their policy at this time. Nevertheless, such experiences have left their mark. Some gays and lesbians reported that they had opted for other therapies, in spite of an interest in psychoanalysis, because they feared rejection (Torelli and Edinger, 1999). Others find themselves in the position of applying and being accepted to less restrictive institutes but then nevertheless being taught theories about the pathology of homosexuality during their training.

University Students

Scientific research in Germany is increasingly accepting studies with gay or lesbian subjects, including student dissertations and theses. However students occasionally worry that the choice of their homosexual subjects constitutes a form of coming out. Some also fear that choosing this subject for their dissertation may lead to discrimination when they apply for jobs (Steffens and Grossmann, 2001).

Professional Organizations

Over the last 25 years, groups dealing with career aspects have been formed, initially by gay men, within the German gay liberation movement. *Schwule Ärzte und Therapeuten Berlin* [Gay Doctors and Therapists Berlin] started on a local level in 1977/78. Then, in 1980, the *Bundesarbeitsgemeinschaft Schwule im Gesundheitswesen* (BASG) [German Association of Gays in the Health Service] was founded followed by the *Verband lesbischer Psychologinnen und schwuler Psychologen in Deutschland e.V.* (VLSP) [Association of Lesbian and Gay Psychologists in Germany] in 1993. These groups represent the interests of professional health workers and organize regular meetings and conferences. The subjects discussed by the study groups have changed since their inception. In the early days, promoting the removal of the diagnosis of Homosexuality from the ICD-9 was part of the national agenda. However, the appearance of AIDS–coping with personal losses and society's attitudes toward the disease–has dominated a significant part of the discussions. At the same time, the policies on training of gay and lesbian professionals, the theories of homosexuality, and issues relating to counseling have been critically examined. The professional groups also offer supervision and Balint groups and discuss relevant current events.

Despite the changed social climate, however, coming out at work reappears on the agenda at regular intervals. Although gays and lesbians are faced with more subtle forms of discrimination at work, it is still necessary to differentiate between their understandable real fears in a society which is still not favorably disposed towards homosexuals and the acceptance of unnecessary concealment and suffering which is often rooted in their own homosexual conflicts (Gooß, 1989). Today there are a number of openly gay or lesbian doctors and psychologists, even an occasional openly gay or lesbian consultant or medical director, who appear to suffer no significant disadvantages because of their homosexuality. Overall, gay and lesbian health workers are nowadays likely to face a range of responses in their professional environments–from still existing pathologization, latent homophobia and heterosexism, to acceptance. There is no question that changes still need to be made.

NOTES

1. At least in its liberalized form with a higher age of consent for male homosexual contacts.

2. Editor's Note: Also See Lauritsen, J. & Thorstad, D. (1974), *The Early Homosexual Rights Movement (1864-1935).* New York: Times Change Press.

3. Editor's Note: For an early "third sex" theory, see Ulrichs, K. (1864), *The Riddle of "Man-Manly" Love,* trans. M. Lombardi-Nash. Buffalo, NY: Prometheus Books, 1994.

4. Editor's Note: See Plant, R. (1986), *The Pink Triangle: The Nazi War Against Homosexuals.* New York: Henry Holt.

5. The heterosexual age of consent of this era actually allowed a man to have intercourse with a girl of 14 if he agreed to marry her. If not, he faced prosecution.

6. Although most West German laws were adopted after the East-West reunification, in the case of homosexuality the East German law prevailed. Since 1994 in Germany, there is only one age of consent (16 years) for both homosexual and heterosexual acts.

7. Editor's Note: In the American tradition, this is usually referred to as "internalized homophobia." See Weinberg, G. (1972), *Society and the Healthy Homosexual.* New York: Anchor Books.

8. Editor's Note: See this issue's interview of Paul Parin regarding Morgenthaler's work.

9. Morgenthaler's theories were initially not published in psychoanalytic journals, but in a textbook by the German sexologist V. Sigusch, whose name is closely linked to the authors of the study *Der gewöhnliche Homosexuelle.* We mention the choice of publication at this point in order to show Morgenthaler's theoretical frame of reference.

10. Morgenthaler does not say whether the conflicts that lead to an accelerated development of the sexual drive are specific. He bases the subsequent steps on this assumption of an accelerated development of the sexual drive.

11. The psychoanalytic literature that followed Morgenthaler's theories mainly emphasizes the autonomy of the homosexual. In the discussions of that time, which were arguing on the basis of social theory, attempts were made to give homosexuality a positive connotation. Within psychoanalytic discussions, Morgenthaler's theories closely follow Kohut's (1971) psychology of the self. In Germany, however, object relations theory had gained a greater influence. Feminist psychoanalysis stressed the question of gender identity. All this may be the reason why Morgenthaler's theory is usually mentioned with respect, but explains why it is not at the centre of current debates.

12. In this context we would like to mention the endocrinologist G. Dörner, whose research possibly represents the most famous German contribution to research into the genesis of homosexuality. Dörner (1980) defined certain mating behavior of male rats as homosexual. According to the results of his research, this behavior correlates to a large extent with insufficient hormone levels that occur at certain stages during the pregnancy of the mother rat. Dörner also deduced direct proposals for the prevention of human homosexuality from his results. This led to a brief intervention by several German sexologists in the mid-eighties. They not only criticized the considerable method-

ological problems of Dörner's theory, but first and foremost also his scandalous notions of a potential treatment. In the end his ideas were of marginal influence.

13. From a formal logical standpoint, the tautology of this formulation is more than obvious. [Editor's Note: For an updated view on Kernberg's evolving position on his structural theories of homosexual development, see Kernberg, O. F. (2002), Unresolved issues in the psychoanalytic theory of homosexuality and bisexuality. *J. Gay & Lesb. Psychother.* 6(1):9-27.

14. Reiche presented his theories at the fiftieth anniversary of the *Deutsche Psychoanalytische Vereinigung* (DPV) [German Psychoanalytical Association].

15. It was published in paperback and was also reviewed by the gay press.

16. This gender identity disorder may very well be the result of a conflict-laden oedipal situation or an earlier stage of development. In a second stage, the prehomosexual boy develops erotic fantasies which are differentiated over a long time that covers the latency period and early adolescence. Friedman provides no specific reasons as to why the second stage of fantasy development follows the first stage of a disturbed gender identity development. The disturbed gender identity of prehomosexual boys does not appear as such in adults because over the course of their development, masculinity and femininity have become represented in a cognitively more complex manner. Erotic fantasies on the other hand are subject to change of function. According to Friedmann, differentiated sexual fantasies are best understood as parts of the core self. The sequence is important here: disturbed gender identity followed on a secondary level by the development of an erotic fantasy.

17. This is the only possible nonpathologizing interpretation of Friedman's theory which states that the primarily disturbed gender identity of the prehomosexual boy no longer affects him as an adult in the same way because of "cognitively more complex representations" of femininity and masculinity, that is, conscious processes during further socialization.

18. The subconscious messages that they do send may contain elements of the "homosexual dynamics" described in much of the earlier psychoanalytic literature. This, however, would be expected as it is impossible to imagine a process of establishing identity which is free from conflict, separation, etc.

19. Because there is a very great number of other treatment modalities available in Germany, and because all other types of psychotherapy have to be financed by the patient, we limit ourselves to the conditions relevant to professionals working in the public health service.

20. This may have been intentional (unpublished data).

REFERENCES

BASG [*Bundesarbeitsgemeinschaft Schwule im Gesundheitswesen*] (1985), *Kritische Glosse: Psychoanalyse in Schwulitäten* [Critical text: Psychoanalysis in difficulty]. *Psyche*, 6:553-560.

Bayer, R. (1981), *Homosexuality and American Psychiatry: The Politics of Diagnosis*. New York: Basic Books.

Benjamin, J. (1988), *The Bonds of Love*. New York: Pantheon Books.

Berger M., ed. (1999), *Psychiatrie und Psychotherapie* [*Psychiatry and Psychotherapy*]. München Wien Baltimore: Urban und Schwarzenberg.

Bergler, E. & Eidelberg, L. (1933), *Der Mammakomplex des Mannes* [The Mother Complex in men]. *Int. Z. Psa.*, 19:555-562.

Bychowski, G. (1961), *Das Ich und das Objekt des Homosexuellen* [The Ego and the object of the homosexual]. *Psyche*, 7:465-474.

Castendyk, S. (1998), *Vom "Objektwechsel" zur Objektwahl* [From "Changing objects" to choosing objects]. *Texte aus dem Colloquium Psycho-analyse*, 3:90-106.

Chasseguet-Smirgel, J. (1975), *L'Idéal du Moi* [*The Ego Ideal: A Psychoanalytic Essay on the Malady of the Ideal*, New York: W. W. Norton, 1985]. Paris: Tchou. [German translation: *Das Ich-Ideal*, 1981].

Chasseguet-Smirgel, J. (1984), *Ethique et Esthétique de la Perversion* [*Ethics and Aesthetics of Perversion*]. Seyssel: Edition du Champ Vallon. [German translation: *Anatomie der menschlichen Perversion*, 1989].

Dannecker, M. (1978), *Der Homosexuelle und die Homosexualität* [*The Homosexual and the Homosexuality*]. Frankfurt/M.: Syndikat.

Dannecker, M. (1990), *Freundlich verpackt. Über R. Isays "Schwul sein"* [Friendly packaging: On Richard Isay's "Being Homosexual"]. *Magnus*, 12:46-47.

Dannecker, M (2000), *Probleme der Männlichen homosexuellen Entwicklung* [Problems of male homosexual development]. *Psyche*, 54:1251-1277.

Dannecker, M. & Reiche, R. (1974), *Der gewöhnliche Homosexuelle* [*The Ordinary Homosexual*]. Frankfurt/M.: Fischer.

Doll, A. (2001), *Berichte an die Gutachter/innen–selbstverständlich lesbisch und schwul?* [Reports to the experts: Lesbian and gay without any question?] In: *Beratung von Lesben und Schwulen* [*Counseling Lesbians and Gays*]. Deutsche Aids-Hilfe e.V., Hg. Berlin: Dt. Aidshilfe e.V., pp. 164-171.

Dörner, G., Geir, T., Ahrens, L., Krell, L., Munx, G., Sieler, H., Kittner, E. & Muller, H. (1980), Prenatal stress as possible aetiogenetic factor of homosexuality in human males. *Endokrinologie*, 75:365-368.

Dörner, K. & Plog, U. (1996), *Irren ist menschlich* [*To Err is Human*]. Bonn: Psychiatrie-Verlag.

Fast, I. (1984), *Gender Identity: A Differentiation Model*. Hillsdale, NJ: The Analytic Press.

Frank, W. (1993), *Kurzlehrbuch zum Gegenstandskatalog mit Hervorhebung und Einarbeitung aller wichtigen Prüfungsfakten* [*Brief Textbook of All the Important Facts for the Exams*]. 11th edition. Neckarsulm Stuttgart: Jungjohann.

Freud, S. (1920), *Über die Psychogenese eines weiblichen Falles von Homosexualität*. In: Freud S.: *Gesammelte Werke*, Bd. XII. Frankfurt: Fischer 1999. [The psychogenesis of a case of homosexuality in a woman. *Standard Edition*, 18:145-172. London: Hogarth Press, 1955.]

Friedman, R. C. (1993), *Männliche Homosexualität* [*Male Homosexuality: A Contemporary Psychoanalytic Perspective*. New Haven/London: Yale University Press. 1988]. Berlin: Springer.

Gebsattel, V. E. von (1929), *Über Fetischismus* [On fetishism]. *Nervenarzt*, 2,8.

Gebsattel, V. E. von (1932), *Süchtiges Verhalten im Gebiet sexueller Verirrungen* [Addictive behavior in the field of sexual aberrations]. *Mschr. Psychiatr. Nervenkrankh* 82:113.

Gebsattel, V. E. von (1950), *Daseinsanalytische und anthropologische Auslösung der sexuellen Perversionen* [Self-analyzing and anthropological triggering of sexual perversions]. *Z. Sexualforschung*, 2:1.

Gehlen, A. (1940), *Der Mensch–Seine Natur und seine Stellung in der Welt* [*Man: His Nature and His Place in the World*]. 10th edition. Auflage, Frankfurt/M.: Fischer.

Giese, H. (1964), *Der homosexuelle Mann in der Welt* [*The Homosexual Man in the World*]. Stuttgart: Enke.

Giese, H., Hg. (1967), *Die sexuelle Perversion* [*The Sexual Perversion*]. Frankfurt/M.: Akademische Verlagsanstalt.

Gissrau, B. (1993), *Die Sehnsucht der Frau nach der Frau* [*The Desire of Woman for Woman*]. Zürich: Kreuz-Verlag.

Gooß, U. (1989), *Zur Situation Schwuler im Gesundheitswesen* [The status of gays in the health service]. In: *Homosexualität & Gesundheit* [*Homosexuality and Health*], U. Gooß & H. Gschwind, Hg. Berlin: Verlag Rosa Winkel, pp. 13-21.

Heinrich, T. & Biechele, U. (1997), *Die psychotherapeutische Versorgung von Lesben und Schwulen. Eine Umfrage der Regionalgruppe Rhein-Neckar* [The psychotherapeutic resources of lesbians and gays: A survey of the Regional Group Rhine-Neckar]. In: *Versteckt und mittendrin* [*Hidden Yet Right in the Middle* (Proceedings of the 4th Congress of VLSP)], M. C. Steffens & M. Reipen, Hg. München Wien: Profil Verlag, pp. 55-63.

Henningsen, F. (1995), *Identifizierung und die Fähigkeit zu lieben. Zwei Fälle männlicher Homosexualität* [Identification and the capacity for love: Two cases of male homosexuality]. *Europäische Psychoanalytische Föderation: Psychoanalyse in Europa*, 53-70.

Isay, R.A. (1990), *Schwul sein. Die psychologische Entwicklung des Homosexuellen* [*Being Homosexual: Gay Men and Their Development*. New York: Farrar, Straus and Giroux, 1989]. München: Piper.

Junkert-Tress, B. & Reister, G. (1995), *Gegenübertragung bei homoerotischer Übertragung* [The countertransference of homoerotic transference]. *Zsch. Psychosom. Med.*, 41:225-240.

Kernberg, O. (1997), *Wut und Haß. Über die Bedeutung von Aggression bei Persönlichkeitsstörungen und sexuellen Perversionen* [*Aggression in Personality Disorders and Perversion*. New Haven: Yale University Press, 1992]. Stuttgart: Klett-Cotta.

Khan, M. (1979), *Alienation in Perversion*. New York: International Universities Press. [German translation: *Entfremdung bei Perversionen*, 1989]

Klein, M. (1932), *Die Psychoanalyse des Kindes* [*The Psychoanalysis of Children*]. München: Kindler.

Kohut, H. (1971), *The Analysis of the Self*. New York: International Universities Press.

Köllner, E. (1994), *Schwul und selbstbewußt* [*Gay and Self-Confident*]. Reinbek: Rowohlt.

Kunz, H. (1942), *Zur Theorie der Perversion* [Toward a theory of perversion]. *Schw. Mschr. Psychiatr. Neurol.*, 105:1.

Kunz, H. (1954), *Zur Frage nach dem Wesen der Norm* [On the question of what is normal]. *Psyche, 6:241.*

Künzler, E. (1991). *Über* "Male Homosexuality. A Contemporary Psychoanalytic Perspective" *von* R. C. Friedman. *ZfSF*, 1:75-80.

Künzler, E. (1992), *Der homosexuelle Mann in Psychoanalyse* [The homosexual man in psychoanalysis]. *Forum Psychoanal.*, 8:202-216.

Le Soldat, J. (2000), *Der Strich des Apelles. Zwei homosexuelle Leidenschaften* [Apelles' stroke: Two homosexual passions]. *Psyche*, 54:742-767.

Mahler, M., Pine, F. & Bergman, A. (1975), *The Psychological Birth of the Human Infant: Symbiosis and Individuation.* New York: Basic Books.

McDougall, J. (1978), *Plaidoyer pour une certaine anormalité* [*Plea for a Measure of Abnormality*. New York: International Universities Press, 1980]. Paris: Gallimard. [German translation: *Plädoyer für eine gewisse Anormalität*, 1989].

Mitchell, S. A. & Aron, L., eds. (1999), *Relational Psychoanalysis: The Emergence of a Tradition.* Hillsdale, NJ: The Analytic Press.

Möller, H.-J. (1995), *Psychiatrie* [*Psychiatry*]. Stuttgart: Hippokrates.

Morgenthaler, F. (1984), *Homosexualität. Heterosexualität. Perversion.* Frankfurt/M/Paris: Qumran. Translated as *Homosexuality Heterosexuality Perversion*, trans. A. Aebi. Hillsdale, NJ: The Analytic Press, 1988.

Poluda-Korte, E. S. (1993), *Der lesbische Komplex* [The Lesbian Complex]. In: *Stumme Liebe* [*Unspoken Love*], E. M. Alves, Hg. Freiburg: Kore.

Rauchfleisch, U. (1993), *Homosexualität und psychoanalytische Ausbildung* [Homosexuality and psychoanalytic training]. *Forum Psychoanal.*, 9:339-347.

Rauchfleisch, U. (2001), *Arbeit im psychosozialen Feld–Beratung, Begleitung, Psychotherapie, Seelsorge* [*Working in the Psychosocial Field: Counseling, Company, Psychotherapy, Pastoral Counseling*] Göttingen: Vandenhoek & Ruprecht.

Reiche, R. (2000a), *Der gewöhnliche Weg zur Homosexualität beim Mann* [The ordinary way to homosexuality in men]. In: *Männlichkeitsentwürfe* [*Sketches of Masculinity*], H. Bosse& V. King, Hg. Frankfurt/M.: Campus, pp. 178-198.

Reiche, R. (2000b), *Die Rekonstruktion der zentralen Onaniephantasie in der Analyse eines jungen Homosexuellen* [The reconstruction of a central masturbation fantasy in the analysis of a young homosexual male]. In: *Sexualität und Gesellschaft* [*Sexuality and Society*], M. Dannecker & R. Reiche, Hg. Festschrift für Volkmar Sigusch. Frankfurt/M.: Campus, pp. 360-383.

Rimmler, U. (1998), *Heterosexismus in der Psychotherapie* [Heterosexism in psychotherapy]. In: *Identitätsbildung, Identitätsverwirrung, Identitätspolitik–eine psychologische Standortbestimmung für Lesben, Schwule und andere* [*Identity Formation, Identity Confusion, Identity Politics: A Psychological Orientation for Lesbians, Gays and Others*]. U. Biechele, Hg. Berlin: DAH e.V, pp. 162-172.

Schelsky, H. (1955), *Soziologie der Sexualität* [*Sociology of Sexuality*]. Reinbek: Rowolt.

Schwarz, O. (1932), *Psychologie des Welterlebens und der Fremdheit* [The psychology of experience and of alienation]. *Z. Neur.*, 139: 97.

Siems, M. (1980), *Coming out–Hilfen zur homosexuellen Emanzipation* [*Coming Out: Assistance for Homosexual Emancipation*]. Reinbek: Rowohlt.

Socarides, C. (1968), *Der offen Homosexuelle* (*The Overt Homosexual*, New York, Grune & Stratton). Frankfurt/M.

Steffens, M. C. & Grossmann, T. (2001), *Forschungsarbeiten über lesbische und schwule Themen* [Scientific research on lesbian and gay topics]. In: *Beratung von*

Lesben und Schwulen [Counseling Lesbians and Gays]. Deutsche Aids-Hilfe e.V., Hg. Berlin: Dt. Aidshilfe e.V., pp. 172-173.

Straus, E. (1930), *Geschehnis und Erlebnis [Happening and Experience]*. Berlin: Springer.

Symalla, T. & Walther, H. (1997), *Systemische Beratung schwuler Paare [Systemic Counseling of Gay Couples]*. Heidelberg: Carl Auer.

Tölle, R. (1999), *Psychiatrie [Psychiatry]*. 12th edition. Berlin, Heidelberg, New York: Springer.

Torelli, M. & Edinger, M. (1999), *Homosexualität–(K)ein Thema in der psychoanalytischen Ausbildung* [Homosexuality–(Non-)topic in psychoanalytic training). In: *Lesben und Schwule in der Arbeitswelt [Lesbians and Gays in the Work World]*, Deutsche Aids-Hilfe e. V., Hg. Berlin: DAH, pp. 174-175.

Wiesendanger, K. (2001), *Schwule und Lesben in Psychotherapie, Seelsorge und Beratung [Gays and Lesbians in Psychotherapy, Pastoral Care and Counseling]*. Göttingen: Vandenhoek & Ruprecht.

Psychiatric, Psychoanalytic, and Mental Health Profession Attitudes Toward Homosexuality in Switzerland

Prof. Dr. Udo Rauchfleisch

SUMMARY. During the past 10 years, theoretical models of homosexuality have changed in Switzerland from a pathological view to one in which homosexuality is a non-pathological orientation equivalent to heterosexuality. Although it is a rarely discussed topic in the professional literature, there is a growing number of courses and lectures about homosexuality in the universities and schools of social sciences in Switzerland. Pathologizing therapists are usually members of religious groups and they are not psychologists and psychiatrists with professional qualifications. In several towns, lesbian and gay therapists are working together in informal groups, and there is a national organization of lesbian and gay therapists called "medy gays." Being openly lesbian or gay still carries great risk for psychiatrists and psychologists who may not be accepted for psychoanalytic training. Swiss Psychoanalytic institutes are reluctant to openly discuss their admission policies. The paper concludes by calling for investigations of the traumatic outcomes of sexual conversion therapies undertaken by fundamentalist religious groups and for more research regarding the situation of older lesbians and gays. *[Article copies available for a fee from The Haworth Document Delivery Service: 1-800-HAWORTH. E-mail address: <getinfo@haworthpressinc.com> Website: <http://www.HaworthPress.com> © 2003 by The Haworth Press, Inc. All rights reserved.]*

Udo Rauchfleisch is Professor of Clinical Psychology, University of Basel/Switzerland and psychotherapist in private practice.

[Haworth co-indexing entry note]: "Psychiatric, Psychoanalytic, and Mental Health Profession Attitudes Toward Homosexuality in Switzerland." Rauchfleisch, Udo. Co-published simultaneously in *Journal of Gay & Lesbian Psychotherapy* (The Haworth Medical Press, an imprint of The Haworth Press, Inc.) Vol. 7, No. 1/2, 2003, pp. 47-54; and: *The Mental Health Professions and Homosexuality: International Perspectives* (ed: Vittorio Lingiardi, and Jack Drescher) The Haworth Medical Press, an imprint of The Haworth Press, Inc., 2003, pp. 47-54. Single or multiple copies of this article are available for a fee from The Haworth Document Delivery Service [1-800-HAWORTH, 9:00 a.m. - 5:00 p.m. (EST). E-mail address: getinfo@haworthpressinc.com].

KEYWORDS. Gay and lesbian therapists, non-pathological model of homosexuality, research in homosexuality, sexual conversion therapy, Swiss psychiatry, Swiss psychoanalysis

If one looks for the prevailing theoretical models about homosexuality in the professional literature in Switzerland, it is difficult to describe a specific Swiss attitude. Since Switzerland is a small country, there are only a few publishers and the number of Swiss scientific articles and books is comparatively small. Most of the psychological and psychiatric journals and psychotherapeutic publications in the German language come from Germany; some are from Austria. Those publications which stand out are by Bochow (1994), Dannecker and Reiche (1974), Gissrau (1993), Künzler (1992a, 1992b), Lautmann (1993), Morgenthaler (1978), Rauchfleisch (1993a, 1993b, 1995, 1994/2001), Wiesendanger (2001) and volume 9/4 (1996) of the journal "System Familie" about counseling and psychotherapy of lesbian and gay individuals and couples.

The theoretical models of homosexuality found in the Swiss professional literature have changed during the past 10 years from a pathological view (i.e., Dorey, 1995) to the model that homosexuality is a non-pathological sexual orientation equivalent to heterosexuality (Dannecker, 2000; Rohde-Dachser, 1994). From my point of view, this shift was provoked by the change of attitudes toward homosexuality in the general society. This change is also the result of the activities of both international and national lesbian and gay movements. Homosexuality is still a rarely-discussed topic in the professional literature. But when it is discussed, the prevailing theoretical model is that of homosexuality as a sexual orientation—which in itself has nothing to do with psychological health or illness—and that it is an orientation equivalent to heterosexuality (Frossard, 2000; Rauchfleisch, 2001; Wiesendanger, 2001).

Topics in psychological and psychiatric publications, for example, deal with discrimination against lesbians and gays in general and with the consequences of such behavior (Rauchfleisch, 2001), with work discrimination (Schneeberger, Rauchfleisch and Battegay, in press), with the concept of homophobia (Hug, 1999; Räss, 1999) and with the extent of homophobia in social professions (Calmbach and Rauchfleisch, 1999), with the essentials of counseling and psychotherapy of lesbians and gays (Frossard, 2000; Wiesendanger, 2001), with problems in the coming out process (Rauchfleisch, 1996, 2001), with the experiences that gay and lesbian patients have had in psychotherapy and counseling (Frossard, 2000; Kämpfer and Fluri, 2000) and comparing the satisfaction of lesbian partnerships with and without children (Krüger-Lebus and Rauchfleisch, 1999). These publications are in the tradition of the earlier literature published by Dannecker and Reiche (1974), Gissrau (1993),

Morgenthaler (1978) and from the German translations of the books of Isay (1990) and Friedman (1993). The authors of these publications argue for a non-pathological concept of homosexuality. Moreover, homosexuality has been increasingly normalized in post-graduate courses in psychiatry, psychology, social work, nursing, and other professions in the social sciences at the Basel and Bern Universities and in different institutions for the training of social workers in other Swiss cities.

The publications, lectures, and other scientific activities concerning homosexuality carried out at the universities in Switzerland are published twice a year in a *Handbook of Lesbian and Gay Studies in Switzerland* (published by "Koordinationsstelle Homosexualität und Wissenschaft, Universität Zürich"). Some notable examples are cited below.

Lectures: 1.11.1996 Psychoanalytisches Seminar Zürich "*Schwules Leben, von einem Analytiker erfahren, erlebt, reflektiert*" ("Gay life, experienced and reflected by a psychoanalyst") by Erhard Künzler (München); 8.4.1998 Bern University "*Sprechen Schwule anders als Heteros?*" ("Do gays speak differently than heteros?") by Jaroslaw Kilian (Basel); lectures in April, May and June 1999 Basel University "*Homosexuelle Orientierungen: Vorurteile and Realitäten*" ("Homosexual orientations: prejudices and realities") by Udo Rauchfleisch; 18.5.2001 Psychoanalytisches Seminar Zürich "*Aids, Sexualität und magisches Denken*" ("Aids, sexuality and magical thinking") by David Signer (Zürich).

Unpublished studies: "*Junge Männer–alte Schwule. Presse- und Polizeiberichterstattung über Gewalt an Schwulen 1958-1990*" ("Young men, old gays. Articles in papers and police reports about violence against gays, 1958-1990") by Erasmus Walser (Bern); "Tony Kushner's Angels in America: Beyond Closet Theatre" by Vitus Gämperli (Zürich); "*Handlungsstrategien bisexueller Frauen*" ("Coping strategies of bisexual women") by Claudia Arnold (Zürich); "*La perception sociale de l'homosexualité masculine*" ("The social perception of male homosexuality") by Sylvie Rochat (Lausanne); "*Lesben und Schwule im Basler Vereinssport*" ("Lesbians and gays in Basel's sportclubs") by Beatrice Calmbach (Basel); "*Homosexuelle Entwicklung in der Pubertät und Adoleszenz*" ("Homosexual development in puberty and adolescence") by Priska Winter and Monika Zürcher (Bern).

As mentioned above, most of the professional literature talks about gay and lesbian clients/patients in a non-pathological way. Generally, those aspects which show great similarities with heterosexual behavior are most exactly perceived by heterosexual therapists. Since these therapists often have little knowledge of the specific difficulties which lesbians and gays experience in their development and with which they are confronted in their present life, such problems are often neglected in therapies (Frossard, 2000). Moreover, in spite of using non-pathological concepts, there are still some publications about mentally ill lesbians and gays where psychic disturbances and homosexuality are causally connected in the sense that homosexuality is interpreted as the expression of psychic illness (Dorey, 1995). But one increasingly finds in the Swiss professional literature that the specific conditions of the development and life of lesbians and gays are presented and discussed. Furthermore, there is quite a lot of interest in this literature among a growing number of professionals in psychology, psychiatry, and social work.

Nevertheless, it is a fact that there is no real discussion between the two "camps pro and contra homosexuality." It is my impression that the minority of psychologists and psychiatrists who regard homosexuality as a sign of psychic pathology do not want to discuss this topic, but just convince the other "camp" to accept the pathological model. On the other hand, the majority of psychologists and psychiatrists who regard homosexuality as an orientation equivalent to heterosexuality are not interested in discussing positions which have finally been repudiated. In addition, most pathologizing therapists are members of religious groups and are not psychologists and psychiatrists with professional qualifications. Therefore it is not possible to have a professional discussion with them.

There are only a few recently published investigations about reports or anecdotal tales about the experience of seeing a mental health provider who knows the patient is gay or lesbian (Frossard, 2000; Wiesendanger, 2001). As these investigations show, therapists who call themselves "open" and "tolerant" often stress the point that there are no differences between heterosexual and homosexual clients. However, this leads the therapists to overlook all the specific conditions of lesbians and gays in our society; for example, using heterosexual marriage as a frame of reference for a same-sex partnership or by neglecting the trauma which many lesbians and gays experience from living in a heterosexist and homophobic society. As the subjects in Frossard's (2000) investigation described their experiences, they felt well understood by their therapists in problems that are not overly influenced by one's sexual orientation. On the other hand, patients/clients often reported that in therapies conducted by heterosexual therapists, they had the "expert status" concerning information about lesbian and gay ways of living. This made the therapy difficult for them, especially when they felt that the therapist in his/her argumentation always starts from a heterosexual frame of reference.

In the larger Swiss cities, for most lesbian and gay clients, it is not difficult to get information (generally from the local lesbian and gay organizations or by lesbian and gay book shops) about therapists who are experienced in treating lesbians and gays. Since Switzerland is quite a small country with comparatively small towns and an open atmosphere concerning homosexuality, lesbian and gay therapists are, in general, known by their colleagues. One consequence of this is that often lesbian and gay clients/patients are sent to these openly lesbian and gay therapists. Moreover, in some towns lesbian and gay therapists are working together in informal groups that are in contact with the local psychological and psychiatric associations. There is also one national organization, "medy gays," a group of lesbian and gay psychologists and psychiatrists. Lesbian and gay clients who look for therapists either get into contact with them through the "medy gays" or they ask for a list of recommended therapists at the local lesbian and gay organizations or the gay book shops of their town. Until now, there have been no publications concerning openly lesbian and gay therapists.

Concerning the relationship between heterosexual colleagues and lesbian and gay therapists, it seems to me that the fact of being lesbian or gay is rarely openly discussed, especially not with the lesbians and gays themselves on an official level. One "knows," but does not talk about "it." It is a type of hypocrisy described by Moor in an article published in 1990. The fact of the therapists' being lesbian or gay is only discussed in private circles.

What is difficult is the situation for psychologists and psychiatrists who want to start training or who are already in training in one of the Swiss psychoanalytic institutes. Being openly lesbian or gay still carries great risk for those professionals as they may not be accepted for psychoanalytic training. In an investigation regarding the admissions policy of the psychoanalytic institutes in Germany, Switzerland and Austria (Rauchfleisch, 1993b) toward openly lesbian and gay colleagues, five of the six Swiss institutes did not answer themselves. Instead, they sent the questionnaire to the president of the Swiss Psychoanalytic Association and she answered, in the name of all these Swiss institutes, "I am sorry to let you know that it is impossible to answer such a complex question."

CONCLUSION

Summarizing the situation in Switzerland, it can be said that in general there is an open and accepting atmosphere toward lesbians and gays. Increasingly, the topic of homosexuality has become part of the curriculum in the Swiss universities and in social work schools. What is still needed in Switzerland are investigations about the following two topics.

First, we need investigations about the outcome of traumatizations by therapists of fundamentalist religious groups. These individuals, who usually do not have any formal therapeutic training and who, based on the theories of Nicolosi, Socarides and Comiskey, try to "heal" lesbians and gays by converting homosexuality to heterosexuality. To date, there are no systematic, detailed studies done in Switzerland that show the impact on lesbians and gays who are currently or have formerly undergone such experiences. There are only anecdotal reports of individuals who suffer from feelings of severe guilt and shame and who become at times suicidal because of the unbearable conflict between their homosexual orientation and the demands of their religious group.

The second topic requiring more research in Switzerland concerns older lesbians and gays. There is a lack of detailed information from large investigations about their situation, their partnerships, their social relations, and the way they live, for example in institutions for the aged. From anecdotal reports, it is known that in such institutions, many lesbians and gays live "closeted." In Zürich, there is a project to create an institution for elderly lesbians and gays called "*Andersheim. Neue Lebens- und Wohnformen, vorwiegend für ältere homosexuelle Männer und Frauen.*" I am also planing an investigation concerning the "gay-and-gray" topic, if possible together with colleagues in Germany and I am in contact with a German institution for aged gays in Köln/Germany, called "*Schwules Seniorenbüro NRW.*"

REFERENCES

Bochow, M. (1994), *Schwuler Sex und die Bedrohung durch Aids–Reaktionen homosexueller Männer in Ost- und Westdeutschland [Gay Sex and the Threat of Aids: Reactions of Gay Men in East and West Germany]*. Berlin: Deutsche Aids-Hilfe.

Calmbach, B. & Rauchfleisch, U. (1999), *Lesbenfeindliche Einstellungen in sozialen Berufen* [Hostile attitudes to lesbians in social professions]. *Wege zum Menschen*, 51:39-45.

Dannecker, M. (2000), *Probleme der männlichen homosexuellen Entwicklung* [Problems of male homosexual development]. *Psyche*, 54:1251-1277.

Dannecker, M. & Reiche, R. (1974), *Der gewöhnliche Homosexuelle [The Ordinary Homosexual]*. Frankfurt/M.: Fischer.

Dorey, R. (1995), *Die Problematik der männlichen Homosexualität. Eine strukturelle Annäherung [The problem of male homosexuality: A structural approach]*. *Europäische Psychoanalytische Föderation: Psychoanalyse in Europa*, 11-33.

Friedman, R.C. (1993), *Männliche Homosexualität [Male Homosexuality: A Contemporary Psychoanalytic Perspective*. New Haven/London: Yale University Press. 1988]. Berlin: Springer.

Frossard, J. (2000), *Lesbische Frauen in der Psychotherapie [Lesbian Women in Psychotherapy]*. Unpublished doctoral dissertation, Basel University.

Gissrau, B. (1993), *Die Sehnsucht der Frau nach der Frau [The Desire of Woman for Woman]*. Zürich: Kreuz-Verlag.

Hug, F. (1999), *Empirische Untersuchungen über Fremd- und Selbsteinschätzungen von Lesben und Schwulen–Implikationen zum Begriff der Homophobie [Empirical Investigation of Self and Other Estimation of Lesbians and Gays: Implications for the Concept of Homophobia*]. Unpublished paper, Dept. of Social Psychology, Bern University.

Isay, R.A. (1990), *Schwul sein. Die psychologische Entwicklung des Homosexuellen* [*Being Homosexual: Gay Men and Their Development*. New York: Farrar, Straus and Giroux, 1989]. München: Piper.

Kämpfer, N. & Fluri, P. (2000), *unbeachtet mittendrin. Diskriminierung von schwulen und lesbischen KlientInnen in der ambulanten Beratung* [*Unnoticed in the Center. Discrimination Against Gay and Lesbian Clients in Ambulatory Counseling*]. Unpublished Diploma Thesis Fachhochschule Zürich–Hochschule für Soziale Arbeit.

Krüger-Lebus, S. & Rauchfleisch, U. (1999), *Zufriedenheit von Frauen in gleichgeschlechtlichen Partnerschaften mit und ohne Kinder* [Satisfaction of women in same sex relations with and without children]. *System Familie*, 12:74-79.

Künzler, E. (1992a), *Der homosexuelle Mann in der Psychoanalyse* [The homosexual man in psychoanalysis]. *Forum Psychoanal.*, 8:202-216.

Künzler, E. (1992b), *Kann ein Homosexueller Psychoanalytiker werden/sein?* [Can a homosexual become/be a psychoanalyst?]. In: *Psychoanalyse im Widerspruch*, ed. Institut für Psychotherapie und Psychoanalyse Heidelberg-Mannheim, Volume 3, pp. 21-38.

Lautmann, R. (1993), *Homosexualität. Handbuch der Theorie- und Forschungsgeschichte* [*Homosexuality. Handbook of the History of Theory and Research*]. Frankfurt/M.: Campus.

Moor, P. (1990), *Homosexualität und psychoanalytische Heuchelei* [Homosexuality and psychoanalytic hypocrisy]. *Psyche*, 44:545-558.

Morgenthaler, F. (1978), *Homosexualität. Heterosexualität. Perversion.* Frankfurt/M.: Fischer Taschenbuch Verlag. Translated as *Homosexuality. Heterosexuality. Perversion,* trans. A. Aebi. Hillsdale, NJ: The Analytic Press, 1988.

Räss, D. (1999), *Drei Instrumente zur Einstellungsmessung von Homophobie* [*Three Instruments for Evaluation of Homophobia*]. Zürich: zart & heftig–Schwules Hochschulforum, Koordinationsstelle Homosexualität & Wissenschaft.

Rauchfleisch, U. (1993a), *Homosexuelle Männer in Kirche und Gesellschaft* [*Gay Men in Church and Society*]. Düsseldorf: Patmos.

Rauchfleisch, U. (1993b), Homosexualität und psychoanalytische Ausbildung [Homosexuality and psychoanalytic training]. *Forum Psychoanal.*, 9:339-347.

Rauchfleisch, U. (1995), *Die stille und die schrille Szene. Erfahrungen von Schwulen im Alltag* [*The Quiet and the Shrill Scene: Experiences of Gays in Everyday Life*]. Freiburg/Br.: Herder.

Rauchfleisch, U. (1996), *Zur Beratung männlicher Adoleszenten mit homosexueller Orientierung und ihrer Eltern* [Counseling of gay adolescents and their parents]. *Prax. Kinderpsychol. Kinderpsychiat.*, 45:166-170.

Rauchfleisch, U. (2001), *Schwule. Lesben. Bisexuelle. Lebensweisen, Vorurteile, Einsichten* [*Gays. Lesbians. Bisexuals. Ways of Living, Prejudices, Insights*]. Third Edition. Göttingen: Vandenhoeck & Ruprecht.

Rohde-Dachser, C. (1994), *Männliche und weibliche Homosexualität* [Male and female homosexuality]. *Psyche*, 48:827-841.

Schneeberger, A., Rauchfleisch, U. & Battegay, R. (in press), *Psychosomatische Folgen und Begleitphänomene der Diskriminierung am Arbeitsplatz bei Menschen mit homosexueller Orientierung* [Psychosomatic effects of discrimination at work for persons with homosexual orientation]. *Schweiz. Arch. Neurol. Psychiat.*

Wiesendanger, K. (2001), *Schwule und Lesben in Psychotherapie, Seelsorge und Beratung* [*Gays and Lesbians in Psychotherapy, Pastoral Care and Counseling*]. Göttingen: Vandenhoek & Ruprecht.

Look to Norway?
Gay Issues and Mental Health
Across the Atlantic Ocean

Reidar Kjær, MD

SUMMARY. This paper addresses the origin of the current theoretical framework for Norwegian psychiatry's understanding of homosexuality. In Norway today, the prevailing attitude is an essentialistic, non-psychopathological understanding of homosexuality based on the generally vague psychosocial and biological understanding of mental health problems and illnesses. This paper points to the influence in Norway of German academic psychiatry, and the impact of both pre- and post-World War II psychoanalytic theories. The gay movement's influence on the pro-gay legislation and position statements in psychiatry is emphasized. Since the radical 1970s, little research has been done in this field of Norwegian psychiatry. This has led to a situation where firm knowledge is scarce and there is a demand for establishing a special competence center. This vacuum has allowed psychoanalysts to fall behind on their theoretical updates and for religious groups to import the reparative therapy movement. Both groups are now challenged. The discrepancy between the pro-gay legislation and the lack of development in

Reidar Kjær is a specialist in psychiatry and works in private practice in Oslo.

Address correspondence to: Reidar Kjær, MD, Postboks 7090 Homansbyen, 0306 Oslo, Norway (E-mail: rekjaer@online.no).

The author wants to thank Mia Berner, Øyvind Ekelund, Jaran Eriksen and Cecilie Rasch-Halvorsen for help and support.

[Haworth co-indexing entry note]: "Look to Norway? Gay Issues and Mental Health Across the Atlantic Ocean." Kjær, Reidar. Co-published simultaneously in *Journal of Gay & Lesbian Psychotherapy* (The Haworth Medical Press, an imprint of The Haworth Press, Inc.) Vol. 7, No. 1/2, 2003. pp. 55-73; and: *The Mental Health Professions and Homosexuality: International Perspectives* (ed: Vittorio Lingiardi, and Jack Drescher) The Haworth Medical Press, an imprint of The Haworth Press, Inc., 2003, pp. 55-73. Single or multiple copies of this article are available for a fee from The Haworth Document Delivery Service [1-800-HAWORTH, 9:00 a.m. - 5:00 p.m. (EST). E-mail address: getinfo@haworthpressinc.com].

10.1300/J236v07n01_05

Norwegian psychiatry is suggested as a possible field of research. *[Article copies available for a fee from The Haworth Document Delivery Service: 1-800-HAWORTH. E-mail address: <getinfo@haworthpressinc.com> Website: <http://www.HaworthPress.com> © 2003 by The Haworth Press, Inc. All rights reserved.]*

KEYWORDS. Gay civil rights, homosexuality, Norwegian psychiatry, position statements, psychoanalysis

If there is anyone who still wonders why this war is being fought, let him look to Norway . . .

And if there is anyone who doubts the democratic will to win, again I say let him look to Norway . . .

Franklin Delano Roosevelt

When US President Franklin D. Roosevelt gave this speech in September of 1942, he wanted to focus on the eager resistance with which the Norwegian resistance movement met the German Nazi invaders.

After World War II, Norway received much support from the US, not least through the Marshall Plan. In the late 1940s, 50s and early 60s, Norway's link to the US was strong in most social and economic areas. An example of this was Norway's joining NATO in 1949. Today there is a focus on another kind of struggle which has links with the US: the fight for equal civil rights for gays and lesbians and the effect of this struggle on the mental health system.

Through legislation, the Norwegian government has increased civil rights for gays and lesbians over the past 30 years. As Norway is one of the most "gay-friendly" nations in the area of civil rights legislation, it raises the interesting question of how does this influence theoretical and clinical psychiatry and what is the actual situation for gays and lesbians concerning mental health services in Norway? This paper provides the historical background necessary to understand the existing situation in Norwegian psychiatry and its relationship to gay and lesbian issues. It also describes some important challenges that need to be solved.

THE EARLY INFLUENCES

Post-W.W. II US psychiatry and psychoanalysis comprise one important root of Norwegian psychiatry related to gay and lesbian issues. Continental German psychiatry–from the mid-nineteenth century onward–and prewar psychoanalytic theory comprise another. Homosexuality became a topic of study in German psychiatry around 1870 with Carl Westphal and Richard von Krafft-Ebing being important contributors. In contrast to earlier theories which named sexual acts rather than individuals, "homosexuality" became a term which defined some innate quality of an individual. German academic psychiatry, with its inclination toward descriptive theories and constitutional psychopathogenesis, was the main theoretical supplier to Norwegian psychiatry before W.W. II. The term "sexual psychopathia" was understood as something deep and unchangeable in a person. One of the leading academic psychiatrists in Norway, Gabriel Langfeldt (1895-1983), held this view and was reluctant to accept psychoanalytic theories of homosexuality.[1] Langfeldt's essentialist position sowed the seeds for a belief that many Norwegian psychiatrists still hold today: homosexuality is something deeply founded in the person and that it is primarily inborn. However, this contemporary essentialistic view is now associated with a non-psychopathological attitude towards homosexuality and the word in use is the Norwegian *legning* meaning sexual orientation.

Just as German psychiatry is one force running through the Norwegian history of psychiatry, the pre- and post-W.W. II waves of psychoanalytic influence represent two other important tendencies. The world's first reference to Sigmund Freud's theories in psychiatry textbooks was in the preface to the 1905 edition of a textbook by Ragnar Vogt (1870-1943) (Alnæs, 1994). This early Freudian praeludium may have prepared the ground for the importation of psychoanalysis into Norway in the 1920s and early 1930s. Professor of psychology Harald Schjelderup (1895-1974), psychiatrists Trygve Braatøy (1904-1953) and Nic. Waal (1905-1960), along with writer Sigurd Hoel (1890-1960), should be mentioned among others who facilitated this process. Their contributions also made psychoanalysis part of the broader intellectual sphere in Norway in the 1930s (Stai, 1954). Many of these pioneers shared "The Dream of the Free Person" (Longum, 1986) and consequently, the question emerges: what significance did psychoanalysis have on the professional attitude towards gays and lesbians in Norway?

Wilhelm Reich (1897-1957), Freud's radical pupil, who had to flee from Nazi Germany, lived in Norway from 1934-39. Literally crossing borders, he seems, though, to have had some "blind spots." When asked to accept a trainee who was known to be homosexual, he answered that he did not want to have anything to do with "such swinishness" (Ollendorff Reich, 1969). Thus, even radical elements within the psychoanalytic movement of the 1930s took a position in relationship to gay and lesbian issues that did not break with a psychopathological view of homosexuality.[2] But alternative thinking about sexuality in the *Journal for Sexual Information* between 1932-34 (Evang, 1947) pointed towards a more modern attitude towards sexuality on the whole. And in their daily life, the radical psychoanalysts may have been quite open-minded and accepting, as illustrated by the vignette about Braatøy below.

Reich had caused a deep problem for the psychoanalytic movement with his increasingly unorthodox ideas and laboratory experiments searching for the origins of life. Reich, as symbol of psychoanalysis, offered a welcome focus for attack from academic psychiatrists, particularly as represented by Langfeldt. The latter formed a bulwark against the new US psychoanalytic influence after 1945. When Reich finally left for the United States on the last ship in August 1939, both friends and enemies were probably relieved. Although his departure might have paved the way for increasing tolerance towards homosexuality from the psychoanalytic movement, when the Norwegians woke up on April 9, 1940 they found themselves occupied by Nazi Germany and the next five years involved a different agenda.

In post-war Norway, the Kinsey reports (Kinsey, Pomeroy and Martin, 1948; Kinsey et al., 1953) had a great impact and were recognized as important challenges to earlier views on sexuality, including views on homosexuality. However, it took quite some time for the effects of the reports to become part of contemporary theory and practice (Kjær, 2001c). In the US, there was a movement in psychiatry of the 1940s and 50s towards a more psychopathological view on homosexuality, and at times even a curious alliance between the profession of psychiatry and the values of the political right during the McCarthy years (Lewes, 1988). Several leading Norwegian psychiatrists stayed in the US during the post-war years. What they brought home from their stays abroad were not only new impulses which challenged the older, German academic constitutional and descriptive psychiatry, but also a conservative psychoanalytic view of homosexuality epitomized by Rado's 1940 critique of Freud's innate bisexuality. When those psychoanalytic theories became part of mainstream Norwegian psychiatry, in the late 1950s and early 1960s, Norwegian psychoanalysis ceased to be a radical movement. Consequently, for many gay men and lesbians, organized psychoanalysis has never been considered a supportive force in changing professional and societal views on homosexuality. Instead, gay men and lesbians had to look elsewhere.

THE GAY LIBERATION MOVEMENT
AND NORWEGIAN LEGISLATION

In 1950, Norway's gay liberation movement organized and modeled itself after the Danish organization of 1948. One of the Danish founders, Helmer Fogedgaard, claims to have coined the term *homofil*, meaning homophile, in 1948. This approach was part of a strategy to focus not only on sexuality, but also on love and emotions (Axgil and Fogedgaard, 1985).

In 1951, the Norwegian gay organization, *Det Norske Forbundet av 1948* [The Norwegian League of 1948], sent a brochure to all Norwegian psychiatrists entitled *"Hva vi vil" [What we want]*. The brochure urged psychiatrists to rethink their psychopathological views. The response, even from progressive psychiatrists, was immense silence–although Ørnulv Ødegaard (1901-86) was one exception. He suggested prosecuting the gay association for their effrontery; however, he got no support from the Health Director (Memo, 1951).

From 1951-53, there ensued a fierce debate in Norway over a proposed change in the penal law of 1902. That law criminalized sexual acts between men and could result in penalties of up to one year in prison.[3] It was particularly an alarm raised about the "seduction of adolescents" that lay behind the proposed change and which prompted psychiatrist Ødegaard[4] to express his concerns about the possibility of the gay movement organizing itself. The gay movement began the struggle against the penal code and the legislative debate came to a halt in Parliament and was not taken up again until 1971.

1957 saw the publication of the first Norwegian book with a non-psychopathological attitude to homosexuality: *Vi som føler annerledes [We Who Feel Differently]* was written under the pseudonym "Finn Grodal" by Øivind Eckhoff (1916-2001) together with Arne Heli (born 1924) (Grodal, 1957). Both were non-professionals and co-founders of *Det Norske Forbundet av 1948.* The text referred to the newer, nonpsychoanalytic professional literature in its appeal for justice and human rights for gays and lesbians. It took almost 20 years before these attitudes entered the psychiatric textbooks (Kjær, 2001c).[5]

Finally, in 1970, the leader of *Det Norske Forbundet av 1948*, Karen-Christine Friele (born 1935), edited a booklet called *§213: Onde eller nødvendighet [§213: Evil or Necessity]* that presented the 1969 Speijer Report from The Netherlands. Based on a more modern perspective, the Dutch report concluded that a conversion to homosexuality via childhood seduction was unlikely, and in 1972 Norway's criminal law and its §213 was changed so that sexual actions between men were no longer considered criminal.[6]

Inevitably, the abolition of criminal penalties for same-sex relationships led to other changes. Another important legislative change was Norway's anti-discrimination law of 1981. It states that discrimination on the base of race, religion, ethnicity, and sexual orientation is illegal. Although the law has rarely been used, some examples of pro-gay convictions exist (Hennum, 2001).

In 1993 a partnership law was passed which gave homosexual couples many of the rights of heterosexual marriages. One exception to the law is its denial to same-sex couples of the right to adopt children, although there is presently an ongoing political debate concerning this issue.

Another current debate centers on the Norwegian State Church. Until recently, the church has been excused from the laws regulating employment discrimination. However, the government wishes to include the church under the regulations. The church still refuses to employ homosexual priests who are living in a committed partnership. And for some church groups, the very existence of the church seems to depend solely on the continuous exclusion of gays and lesbians (Moxnes, 2001). In fact, these Norwegian groups have imported the arguments made by American antihomosexual organizations like the National Association for Research on Homosexuality (NARTH) and other religious conversion or "ex-gay" programs (see Dreyfuss, 1999; Shidlo, Schroeder and Drescher, 2001). As in the US, the religious opposition of these groups to gay rights legislation has been increasingly couched in clinical, medical and scientific terms. In many of the official documents connected with laws protecting gay and lesbian civil rights, it has been difficult to find a precise theory of homosexuality. Instead, they refer to *homofili* as a *legning* [sexual orientation] which is something essential. To understand and respond to the clinical theories of antihomosexual political forces, we must turn to the official psychiatric documents for a more developed theoretical framework regarding homosexuality.

NORWEGIAN PSYCHIATRIC ASSOCIATION'S 1977 POSITION STATEMENT

Following the 1972 abolition of Norway's criminal law, young psychiatrists were influenced by events that occurred in the American Psychiatric Association during 1972 and 1973. That was when homosexuality was removed as a diagnosis from the *Diagnostic and Statistical Manual* (Bayer, 1981). Psychiatrists Astrid Nøklebye Heiberg (born 1936) and Helge Waal (born 1940, and the son of Nic. Waal) were the leading professionals who, in collaboration with *Det Norske Forbundet av 1948* and its powerful leader Karen-Christine Friele, worked towards effecting change. Leading up to the time of the Norwegian Psychiatric Association's annual meeting of 1977, there were several discussions on homosexuality in which the participants could roughly be divided into three groups. They included (1) the "young radicals" who favored a non-pathological view of homosexuality; (2) their opponents represented by members of the Norwegian Psychoanalytic Association who held that homosexuality was pathological; and (3) a broader group consisting of psychiatrists who had not yet made up their minds. These three groups of psychiatrists held such different views and attitudes towards homosexuality that the idea of producing a single document upon which they could agree represented quite a challenge. Consequently, the 1977 annual meeting produced a long and complex position statement. Its most important conclusion was that the Norwegian Psychiatric Association recommended that *homofili* (homosexuality) should no longer be used as a psychiatric diagnosis (Kjær, 2001c). This later led to the removal of the diagnosis from the Norwegian version of the *International*

Classification of Diseases (ICD), which still is the official diagnostic system in Norway. But what kind of decision was this? And which theoretical views of homosexuality can be inferred from this statement?

The text uses, a bit inconsistently, both the Norwegian term *homofil*, translated as homophilia, and *homoseksualitet*, translated as homosexuality. The Norwegian term *homofile*, meaning homophile persons, are here translated as homosexuals:

> Homophilia/homosexuality is a description of a special form of sexual behavior or orientation. We will here neither discuss possible causes nor give an evaluation of homosexuality as a positive or negative way of life. This because it is obvious that among psychiatrists there are different opinions on homosexuality.

In Norway in the 1970s, debates between behavioral and psychodynamic theorists were rather fierce. The statement did not take a stand in this matter. It also avoided the ongoing controversy between psychoanalytic and more biological views concerning causality. In this respect, the statement seems to have been a pragmatic one, aiming at reaching a consensus rather than offering a real theoretical framework for psychiatric research and clinical practice.

> Quite a number of homosexuals say that they are satisfied with their sexual orientation. They show no clear psychopathology and their social function is adequate. Other homosexuals are bothered by and in conflict with their sexual orientation. Or they wish to change it. Some seek treatment because of social pressure in society. Psychiatric treatment with the aim of changing sexual orientation seems to have limited chances to succeed. However, if the person seeking help has a strong personal wish for a change there is no doubt that treatment in some cases can give results.

Obviously, the above part of the statement did not support stopping the practice of therapies aimed at changing sexual orientation. From the statement, we must conclude that such therapies were conducted in 1977 and the authors of the position statement needed to get all groups of psychiatrists to vote for it.[7]

> In the debate on psychiatry's attitude towards homosexuality, people often tend to mix different questions together. One topic relates to social discrimination, the next to the use of psychiatric diagnosis and the third to scientific matters.

> Psychiatrists have–like everyone else–an obligation to protest against every unjust discrimination whether it is directed towards homosexuals or others. We want to express our support to homosexuals fighting

against discrimination. Psychiatrists should also not be moralistic when homosexuals come for treatment. The therapist must, together with the patient, clarify the actual situation and background for the problems. This will often imply helping the homosexual patient to accept his or her homosexuality as part of the total identity.

This part of the statement came from the radical "wave," which used ethical standards to take sides with the patient in a societal struggle. The statement used the term "total identity," which may have reflected an essentialistic view of homosexuality. It also favored equal civil rights for gays and lesbians.

Diagnosis or classifications are necessary for every professional communication. But medical diagnoses are not always logically constructed, and are often influenced by historical developmental processes. As psychiatrists we are skeptical about the use of diagnostic classifications in non-professional situations. An example of this can be seen when the diagnosis of hysteria or psychopathy is used in daily life conversations and in public debate. Psychiatric diagnosis has traditionally been used when extensive symptoms or evident deviant personality traits are present. Even though it has been a growing tendency that psychiatric diagnosis has been used to describe behavior and symptoms that earlier would have been regarded as normal, we will state that it is dubious to use psychiatric diagnosis on isolated aspects of behavior. Ideally psychiatric diagnosis should be related to causality in a broader meaning, a broader spectrum of suffering behavior, lowered social functions and/or a wish for treatment. Considering this, it is regarded as unjust to use the term homophilia/homosexuality as a psychiatric diagnosis. We will therefore towards the Health Directory and towards our colleges recommend that homophilia/homosexuality no longer be used as a psychiatric diagnosis.

By omitting any scientific discussion about the possible causes of homosexuality, the statement's authors avoided debates that probably would have made it impossible to agree upon the statement.[8] However, a patient's "wish for treatment" alone made it difficult to justify the use of a psychiatric diagnosis. By refusing to take a stand concerning the causality of homosexuality, the statement's successful arguments for discarding the diagnosis were to be found in the terms "suffering" or "lowered social functioning." By this they may have meant that these qualities were not evident to such a degree that homosexuality could be viewed as a psychiatric illness requiring a diagnosis.

But what about homosexuals who do seek help because of doubt or anxiousness about being homosexual and where this can not directly be ascribed to either discrimination or social pressure and who wants to change their behavior or sexual orientation? Regarding our criteria, these people experience a subjective suffering and need treatment. But even here we do not consider it necessary to use homosexuality as a diagnosis.

As it is difficult to imagine being gay in the 1970s and *not* feeling uncomfortable about it without any direct connection to discrimination or social pressure, this part of the statement seems to indicate a concession to those colleagues who did not support the more radical group of psychiatrists.

Research has produced some knowledge about homosexuality, but we have to admit that our knowledge is insufficient, especially because there has been no access to representative groups of homosexuals. We want to emphasize that research on homosexuality as a social phenomenon is important, among other reasons because lack of knowledge often contributes to prejudice and discrimination.

This part of the statement may represent a possible revolt against a research tradition, embodied in the work of US psychiatrist and psychoanalyst Irving Bieber (Bieber et al., 1962). Bieber's theoretical arguments were used to support a psychopathological view of homosexuality during the debate prior to the annual meeting (Jørstad, 1977). Here the statement takes a firm stand against what were by then already outdated data and ends with the following:

The Norwegian Psychiatric Association wants to emphasize that this position statement does not say whether homosexuality is "as valuable" or "as normal" as heterosexuality. What we do when we recommend that homophilia/homosexuality no longer be used as a diagnosis, is that we as professionals recognize that homophilia itself does not qualify as a psychiatric diagnosis. We also want to emphasize that this position statement must not be interpreted in a way that homosexuals should avoid seeking psychiatric or psychological help if they experience problems. Psychiatrists have treated homosexuals and they will continue to do so. The treatment must then of course be done on the patient's terms.

AFTER 1977: THE LACK OF FOLLOW-UP AND PSYCHIATRIC TEXTBOOKS

Despite the complexity of the position statement of 1977, the only recommendation which was immediately followed up on was that of no longer using the diagnosis of homosexuality. There were no research projects; there were no deeper professional discussions about homosexuality and sexuality; nor was there any improvement in the education of medical student or specialists on the subject of homosexuality. In fact, since issuing the 1977 statement, Norwegian psychiatrists seem to have shown little interest in homosexuality as a professional topic. The number of medical articles have been few and psychiatric textbooks have added limited and little new research since 1977. However, there is one change noticeable in the textbooks: the slow and gradual removal of old research, references and passages which display antihomosexual prejudice or stereotypes about homosexuality. The best example of this is found in the textbooks by one of Norway's leading and most outspoken psychiatrists today, Einar Kringlen (born 1931). The latest editions of his textbook have been edited over the years to such an extent that there is hardly any substantial text left. Even the addition of a few modern references has not made the text suitable to provide students an adequate introduction to knowledge on homosexuality.

From 1971 to 1984, in the textbooks of Leo Eitinger (1912-1995) and Nils Retterstøl (born 1924), one finds a greater understanding and willingness to include more positive evaluations of homosexuality. Parts of these texts originated directly from brochures made by the gay movement, and they were presented in the textbooks without references to the origin. This may support the hypothesis that views first claimed or put forward by the gay movement later become a part of common attitudes among the more humanistically oriented psychiatrists (Kjær, 2001c).

A Swedish textbook that is frequently used in Norway also needs mentioning. The Swedish psychiatrist and psychoanalyst Johan Cullberg (born 1934) has, since 1984, been the author of the popular *Dynamisk Psykiatri [Dynamic Psychiatry]*. His chapter on homosexuality has primarily been based on Irving Bieber's 40-year old findings and conclusions[9] (Kjaer, 2001c). Cullberg has now rewritten his chapter, and states in a remarkably open way that his earlier writing on homosexuality had been influenced by heteronormativity. He also points to the lack of consensus regarding psychodynamic theories and homosexuality and suggests these theories should not be used before a better consensus is achieved (Cullberg, 2001). This makes Cullberg the first leading Scandinavian psychoanalyst to take into account the critiques raised against traditional psychoanalysis and its pathologizing view of homosexuality. This may represent the beginning of an important turn in the Scandinavian psychoanalytic movement similar to the one seen in the US about ten years ago (Isay, 1996).

A GROWING NEW INTEREST IN THE MENTAL HEALTH OF GAYS AND LESBIANS

It was first with the now-famous Norwegian NOVA report pointing to the fact that young gay people have an increased risk of suicidal attempts that an increased focus was directed toward the mental health of gays and lesbians (NOVA, 1999). For example, in the year 2000, Norwegian television showed a film about a young gay Christian boy who had disappeared and most probably committed suicide after joining a charismatic Christian group with strong antihomosexual attitudes. As in other countries, many of the problems that the gay adolescent faces in Norway are related to the difficult coming-out process in a society where heterosexism and antihomosexual attitudes prevail.[10] I have described their psychological situation elsewhere as being like "inner refugees" (Nilsen, 2001).

Recently there has been increasing concern among Norwegian psychiatrists about the effect of the US "reparative treatment" movement, represented by NARTH, and its influence in some Norwegian professional circles. In 1999, after an original initiative by this author, a statement against reparative therapy was put forward at the General Assembly of the Norwegian Psychiatric Association. It was declined and sent back to the board for further review (Kjær, 2001c). In October 2000, the General Assembly voted overwhelmingly (about 90%) in favor of the following statement, using the term "homofili" for homosexuality:

> Homosexuality is no disorder or illness, and can therefore not be subject to treatment. A 'treatment' with the only aim of changing sexual orientation from homosexual to heterosexual must be regarded as ethical malpractice, and has no place in the health system.
>
> Homosexuals have, as everyone else, of course, a right to get help and treatment that follows recommended guidelines, whether this is related to their sexuality or not.

One reason why such a statement was put forward was to counter religious groups seeking support from the psychiatric profession in their charismatic efforts to change sexual orientation through "treatment." This statement is an ethical one, and makes reference to the Hippocratic oath's dictum to do no harm to a patient. While admitting that it is not yet scientifically proven that such an effort is harmful, it does consider such attempts unethical. This is in accordance with the American Psychiatric Association's (APA's) position statements of 1998 and 2000 on reparative or sexual conversion therapies.

As this paper is being written in the fall of 2001, there is an ongoing political debate in Norway about the "religious healing" of gays. Some politicians have referred to the unpublished findings presented by Robert Spitzer in May 2001 at the annual meeting of the APA. Spitzer's study claims that a few of the people who say they have changed sexual orientation, may seem to have done so. The debate on the possible scientific value of this report has yet to be concluded, but the fundamental questions about method and ethical standards have been raised.[11]

The Spitzer findings were used in the Parliamentary discussion when a report from the government to the parliament, *Stortingsmelding nr. 25*, about the health and quality of life situations for lesbians and gays, was discussed on May 31, 2001. The report raises substantial questions about the current health care situation for gays and lesbians, but offers no real answer to this article's search for a theoretical framework. To find such a framework, we seem only to have the statements from 1977 and 2000 and some hints in textbooks. What emerges is a vague, essentialistic non-psychopathological view on homosexuality with very insufficient knowledge available to the clinicians, trainees and medical students in the Norwegian health services. Therefore it has been recommended that a resource center–and possibly also a clinical unit–be established as soon as possible in connection with the University of Oslo where the psychiatric profession can be updated to offer adequate services to gays and lesbians (Kjær & Selle, 2001).

NORWEGIAN PSYCHOANALYTIC ASSOCIATION

Another current, but smaller field of controversy surrounds the Norwegian Psychoanalytic Association. The 1991 change in the American Psychoanalytic Association's attitude towards gay and lesbian professionals wanting to become psychoanalysts (Roughton, 1995) has not yet been repeated here. The Norwegian Psychoanalytic Association is not yet willing to clarify their views, nor have they dismissed their earlier theories of homosexuality as being caused by a certain arrest of psychosexual development (Freud, 1935). This attitude has now been challenged (Kjær and Selle, 2001). We can therefore hope that Norway will now enter a turning point in time, and that what Richard Isay has described can come to life here (Isay, 1996). Isay, a central figure in effecting change in the US, came to Norway in 2000 and held a seminar inspiring the effort now directed towards the Norwegian Psychoanalytic Association. The Association is small, but powerful because they educate people who in turn become educators for therapists.[12] *Landsforeningen for Lesbisk and homofil frigjøring* [National Organization for Lesbian and Gay Liberation] recently gave its annual Homophobia award to the Norwegian Psychoanalytic Association (Kjær, 2001a).[13] However, as many members of the Norwegian Psychoanalytic Association privately express a divergent view, there is hope that in the near future the organization will show a more gay-friendly attitude.

CLINICAL EXPERIENCE OF GAYS AND LESBIANS

The absence of follow-up on the 1977 position statement becomes strikingly visible when one tries to search the professional literature for descriptions of the subjective clinical experience of gays and lesbians. Such expressed subjective experiences were almost non-existent prior to the NOVA report in 1999. One exception to this is a personal report from a lesbian who was hospitalized in 1978. It shows that homosexuality was a "non-topic" on the ward. She was expected to "show" her feelings and "work" with them, but found it difficult at the same time to "calm down" her probably most important feelings (Enderud, 1991).

In the absence of data, this paper will provide some data from the NOVA report which can at least shed some light on the situation in Norway. However, to complete the picture it has to rely upon anecdotes. This of course shows something quite striking about the current situation in Norway. The country has some of the most pro-gay legislation in the world and also the aforementioned position statements advocating non-psychopathological attitudes. But the field of psychiatry has not yet initiated any debate or research or made any educational effort to improve mental health services for this minority. The exception to this is the program of suicide prevention that the NOVA report launched, but which is just in the starting phase.

The NOVA report is a sociological survey which recruited its subjects by advertising in the gay milieu. It suffers for this reason from methodological limitations. In a small chapter called "The Meeting with the Treatment System," it reports that gays and lesbians tend to hold back any information that can identify them as "homosexuals" out of fear of negative reactions which could lead to a qualitatively poorer treatment. The report quotes a new textbook in general medicine which emphasizes that the general practitioner should ask openly about family relations and partners in a way that allows a gay patient to be open and undisguised about his or her situation. A report about lesbians and their experiences in psychological treatment is cited which indicated that therapists, only to a small degree, have been able or willing to see lesbians as a minority group. Taboo topics associated with lesbianism were under-communicated in the treatment relationship where the client was lesbian and the therapist was heterosexual (NOVA, 1999).

Not only is the written material on the clinical experiences of gays and lesbians scarce, unfortunately the well of anecdotes is rather dry. Norwegians are regarded as people who preferably avoid talking about difficult issues in general, and about stigmatized sexuality in particular. An illustrative "slip of the pen" recently occurred in a major Christian hospital in Oslo. A young man with a moderate depression and some "deviant personality traits" was transferred to another hospital because of a change of address. In the medical record accompanying the patient, the assistant resident had written, co-signed by the chief psychiatrist, that there were "no previous illnesses, apart from homosexuality" (Selle, 2001).

At the same hospital, a young gay man on the emergency ward was told that he could pray to God to get rid of his homosexuality, and that this had helped many people before. This recommendation was made by a psychiatric nurse, although it is not known whether this was sanctioned by the psychiatrist in charge. However, the nurse's suggestion took place in a professional climate where she must have understood that such an offering, if not sanctioned, would not be criticized by her superiors.

Another anecdote involves a lesbian who had been in psychotherapy for seven years without the therapist ever knowing that she was a lesbian and living with another woman. The fear of adverse reactions from the therapist is one part of this story, professional scotoma and antihomosexual bias are others.

In the 1930s, a famous Norwegian actor and beloved teller of fairy tales became a friend of the psychiatrist Trygve Braatøy. He wanted to have a consultation about his homosexuality in Braatøy's office, which was granted a bit reluctantly since they were friends. In his autobiography *From My Queer Corner*, the actor gives a vivid description of their professional meeting (Bang-Hansen, 1985):

> I spoke out. Told him bits and pieces about myself. Without hesitation. Finally he was laughing, lying under the table. (One should not laugh at the patients). From the floor he shouted up to me:
>
> Would you like any changes?
>
> No, I shouted back.
>
> This was to be the first and only consultation.

In the field of literature, 2000 saw the publication of a biography of Gunvor Hofmo (1921-1995) one of Norway's leading modernist poets (Vold, 2000). She was for many years a patient in a mental hospital and was diagnosed with paranoid schizophrenia. During W.W. II, she fell in love with a woman, Ruth Maier, a Jew who was sent to Auschwitz and killed there. Hofmo never recovered from the loss and her poems show distance to humans and a strong expression of lost love. Her 1946 book, *I Want to Return to the Human Beings*, is an illustration both of her loss and her illness. She later lived for some years with another woman, but spent her last years alone and isolated in her home. Even today, her biographer, a leading contemporary poet, does not dare to tell the true story about her lesbian love in fear of what her living nephews and nieces might say. In 1953, she proclaimed openly that she was a lesbian and tried to use men's clothes in the hospital. The psychiatrists forced her to wear a dress, and she was reported to "have lost the old spiritual look in her eyes" (Lindstad,

2001). From this we could easily imagine how the loss of her loved one might have been a "non-topic" in the mental hospital as well.

To repeat, these anecdotes show that little is known about the clinical experiences of gays and lesbians either in the professional literature or how they experienced their encounters with the mental health care system. The need for further research is obvious.

OPENLY-GAY AND LESBIAN MENTAL HEALTH PROFESSIONALS

What of the status of openly gay and lesbian mental health professionals in Norway? From personal experience, the reaction is that people meet you with a sort of silent acceptance. Coming out more openly as a gay psychiatrist and having worked on the refused position statement of 1999, I was greeted by a very outspoken young psychiatrist with the following quote: "I really thought your position statement [against reparative therapy] was like kicking in open doors, until I read the report from the annual meeting. Then I saw that the statement is necessary because of all these old fashioned thoughts that are still in circulation."

At the moment, I find the following to be a typical reaction from the majority of heterosexual Norwegian psychiatrists: At best they will direct focus away from you as a gay individual and turn the conversation to professional issues on homosexuality. But that may very well be the constructive path to take. They are, if not gay-friendly, at least gay-neutral and not fully aware of the work that needs to be done in the years to come. Nevertheless, I am certain that it is possible without much difficulty to improve the mental health care system and professional training and offer better mental care for gays and lesbians. However, to accomplish this, the situation for medical students and trainees needs to be more open and accepting.

CONCLUSIONS

The struggle for equal civil rights for gays and lesbians has in many countries been hard and is still ongoing. In Norway, one could imagine that this battle has been won. Anti-discrimination laws, partnership laws, pending adoption rights and also the position statements by the Norwegian Psychiatric Association seemingly offer ideal conditions for gays and lesbians. Research and improvement in clinical practice and education however, do not yet match the formal standards. This discrepancy is suggested as a possible field of research.

One important conclusion can be drawn from this: formal and legislative rights and privileges are of great importance and well worth fighting for. By first winning the battle formally, the ground is secured and prepared for further growth. Psychiatrists and other mental health professionals may be able to safeguard this and also participate in a professional process to improve this situation and thereby the mental health services for all.

Although the civil rights battle in the US has not yet formally been won to the same extent as it has here in Norway, massive research has been done in the US over the last twenty years. This accumulated knowledge opens the possibility for comparative research projects, and there is little doubt that scientific data and US know-how would be very welcome as part of a "Gay Marshall Plan" for Norway. However when it comes to political willingness and possibility to win the fight for gay and lesbian civil rights, I suggest that the reader lend an ear to Franklin D. Roosevelt's appeal and take a closer "Look to Norway."

NOTES

1. Langfeldt was eventually influenced, in part, by the theories of the American psychiatrist and psychoanalyst Irving Bieber (Bieber et al., 1962). Bieber had emphasized the importance of a strong mother-son relationship in fostering the development of male homosexuality (Kjær 2001c).

2. Editor's Note: The German homophile movement of Reich's time was led by Magnus Hirschfeld, a former member of the International Psychoanalytic Association and an advocate of a normal variant view of homosexuality. See Lauritsen, J. & Thorstad, D. (1974), *The Early Homosexual Rights Movement (1864-1935)*. New York: Times Change Press.

3. When the law was first debated in the Parliament, it was suggested that it should also include same sex acts between women. But lesbianism was so unimaginable in 1902 Norway that women were not covered by the law. This may be a rare but positive effect of the usual marginalization and invisibility of lesbians (Rian, 2001).

4. Ødegaard also advocated for castration as a suitable treatment for homosexuals, if they volunteered. In many ways, like US psychiatrist Edmund Bergler, he represented the most outspoken antihomosexual attitudes within psychiatry (Kjær, 2001c).

5. A second book by Eckhoff and Heli, *De tause taler ut [The Silent Speak Up]* consisted of letters written to "Finn Grodal" in reaction to the previous book. This unique documentation of the lives of gay people in the 1950s was submitted for publication, but refused. The manuscript has recently been discovered and is now in preparation for publication.

6. Friele is often credited with winning this second round in the legislative battle which led to the abolition of the penal law (Kjær, 2001c).

7. Editor's Note: A similar compromise took place in the United States in 1973 when the DSM-II's diagnosis of "homosexuality" was replaced by "sexual orientation disturbance." The new diagnosis acknowledged that some individuals were unhappy with their sexual orientation and might seek psychiatric treatment to change it. However, the new diagnosis, because it was a political compromise, also allowed that some

heterosexual individuals might want to change their orientation to homosexuality. Since this was an extremely rare–perhaps nonexistent–clinical phenomenon, sexual orientation disturbance was changed to "ego-dystonic homosexuality" in the 1980 DSM-III. By 1987, the political climate had changed tremendously and ego-dystonic homosexuality was deleted from the DSM-III revision or DSM-III-R.

8. It should be further noted that in those years, the gay movement itself was very eager not to support any kind of causality research. This was based on the fear that if a cause was found, treatment to change sexual orientation could then be developed. They also pointed out that the cause of heterosexuality was never questioned.

9. For some reason, Cullberg has continuously misspelled "Bieber" as "Biber."

10. Criticism is now also increasingly being drawn toward the difficult situation for gays and lesbians outside the major cities of Norway (Mortensen, 2001). In 2000, a local preacher outside the city of Bergen compared gays to pigs on a radio show. His conclusion was that pigs know best because they stick to "The Order of Nature." The preacher, Rev. Flåten from *Livets Ord* [The Words of Life], was reported to the police. However, the *Riksadvokat* [National Attorney] declined to prosecute the case. This was in contrast to his own suggestion of using the anti-discrimination law from 1981 more aggressively after racists, probably neo-nazis, murdered a boy of color in January 2001. When a gay man was hacked to death a few years earlier, there was no mention of using that law more aggressively. Perhaps when hate-crimes are considered, gays tend to come on the bottom part of the list. Society easily forgets that racism, anti-Semitism, anti-homosexual attitudes and discrimination all have similar roots (Kjær, 2001d).

11. Spitzer has tried, unsuccessfully, to warn people from using the report to deny gay and lesbian civil rights. However, he can hardly have been oblivious to the fact that people telling him their stories over the phone could easily manipulate such an easily constructed and non-verifiable survey (Kjær 2001b).

12. Given the comparatively vivid interest in psychodynamic theories and practice in Norway, one could have expected a more numerous organization. However most Norwegian therapists are members of a more open and eclectic milieu, centered around the Institute for Psychotherapy. It could be presumed that most of them share a non-psychopathological, essentialistic view of homosexuality, but research is lacking to confirm this.

13. At the same time, the minister Bekkemellem Orheim, herself a heterosexual, was given the Gay Pride Award for her support of gay issues. She declared herself proud to be called "Gay Minister."

REFERENCES

Alnæs, R. (1994), Psykoanalysen i Norge [The Psychoanalytic Movement in Norway]. *Nord J Psychiatry*, 48 (suppl. 32), 9.

American Psychiatric Association (1998), Position statement on psychiatric treatment and sexual orientation. *Amer. J. Psychiat.*, 1999, (156):1131.

American Psychiatric Association (2000), Commission on Psychotherapy by Psychiatrists (COPP): Position statement on therapies focused on attempts to change sexual orientation (Reparative or conversion therapies). *Amer. J. Psychiat.*, (157):1719-1721.

Axgil, A. & Fogedgaard, H. (1985), *Homofile kampår. Bøsseliv gjennom tidene [Years of Homophile Fighting. Gay Life Through History]*. Rudkøbing: Forlaget Grafolio.

Bang-Hansen, A. (1985), *Fra mitt skjeve hjørne [From My Queer Corner]*. Oslo: Gyldendal.

Bayer, R. (1981), *Homosexuality and American Psychiatry: The Politics of Diagnosis.* New York: Basic Books.

Bieber, I., Dain, H., Dince, P., Drellich, M., Grand, H., Gundlach, R., Kremer, M., Rifkin, A., Wilbur, C. & Bieber T. (1962), *Homosexuality: A Psychoanalytic Study.* New York: Basic Books.

Cullberg, J. (2001), *Dynamisk Psykiatri [Dynamic Psychiatry]*. Stockholm: Natur och Kultur.

Dreyfuss, R. (1999), The holy war on gays. *Rolling Stone*, March 18, pp. 38-41.

Enderud, K. (1991), Søkelys på psykiatrien [Focus on Psychiatry]. *Tidsskriftet Løvetann*, 5, 15.

Evang, K. (1947), *Seksuell opplysning [Information on Sexuality]*. Oslo: Tiden norsk forlag.

Freud, S. (1935), Anonymous (Letter to an American mother). In: *The Letters of Sigmund Freud*, ed. E. Freud, 1960. New York: Basic Books, pp. 423-424.

Grodal, F. [Eckhoff, Ø] (1957), *Vi som føler annerledes [We Who Feel Different]*. Oslo: Aschehoug.

Hennum, R. (2001), Lesbiske og homofiles rettstilling [Law status for gays and lesbians]. In: *Norsk Homoforskning [Gay Science in Norway]*, eds. M. Brantsæter, T. Eikvam, R. Kjær & K. O. Åmås. Oslo: Universitetsforlaget, pp. 85-103.

Isay, R. (1996), *Becoming Gay: The Journey to Self-Acceptance.* New York: Pantheon.

Jørstad, J. (1977), Homoseksualitet hos menn [Homosexuality in men]. *Fokus på familien [Focus on the Family]*, Særtrykk, 1.

Kinsey, A., Pomeroy, W. & Martin, C. (1948), *Sexual Behavior in the Human Male.* Philadelphia, PA: Saunders.

Kinsey, A., Pomeroy, W., Martin, C. & Gebhard, P. (1953), *Sexual Behavior in the Human Female.* Philadelphia, PA: Saunders.

Kjær, R. (2001a), Går tingene sin skjeve gang i norsk psykoanalytisk forening? [How queer is the Norwegian Psychoanalytic Association?] *Tidsskriftet Løvetann* 2, 4-6.

Kjær, R. (2001b), Intoleranse med statsstøtte [Intolerance financed by the government]. *VG* [An important Norwegian daily newspaper] 24, July.

Kjær, R. (2001c), Seksualpsykopaten som forsvant. Homofili i norske psykiatriske lærebøker [The sexual psychopath who disappeared. Homosexuality in Norwegian psychiatry textbooks]. In: *Norsk Homoforskning [Gay Science in Norway]*, eds. M. Brantsæter, T. Eikvam, R. Kjær & K. O. Åmås. Oslo: Universitetsforlaget, pp. 104-140.

Kjær, R. (2001d), Skal vi bygge sammen? Kronikk [Shall we build together? Chronicle], *Dagens Medisin [Medicine Today]*, 16.

Kjær, R. & Selle, M. S. (2001), Levekår og livskvalitet for lesbiske og homofile. Informativ stortingsmelding med utfordringer til helsevesenet [Life situation and quality of life for gays and lesbians. Informative governmental report that challenges the Health Services]. Tidsskrift for den Norske Lægeforening [*J. Norwegian Med. Assn.*], 121, 1884.

Lewes, K. (1988), *The Psychoanalytic Theory of Male Homosexuality*. New York: Simon and Schuster.

Lindstad, S. (2001), Livslang kjærlighetssorg [Life long grief of love]. *Blikk*, februar [2]:46-48.

Longum, L. (1986), *Drømmen om det frie menneske [The Dream of the Free Person]*. Oslo: Universitetsforlaget.

Memo (1951), Memo in the office of the Health Director, 18, December 1951. *Riksarkivet [The Norwegian National Archive]*: Pa 1216 Det norske Forbundet av 1948.

Mortensen, E. (2001), Å leve som seksuell flyktning i sitt eget land [Living as a sexual refugee in one's own country]. *Samtiden* 3:74-81.

Moxnes, H. (2001), Fra kulturelt hegemoni til ideologisk ghetto. Homofili-debatten i den norske kirke fra 1950-2000 [From cultural hegemony to ideological ghetto. The debate on homosexuality in the Norwegian Church 1950-2000]. In: *Norsk Homoforskning [Gay Science in Norway]*, eds. M. Brantsæter, T. Eikvam, R. Kjær & K. O. Åmås. Oslo: Universitetsforlaget, pp. 57-84.

Nilsen, L. (2001), Overser homofiles lidelser [The mental health problems of gays and lesbians are overlooked]. Interview of this article's author in *Dagens Medisin [Medicine Today]* 16.

NOVA (1999), *Levekår og livskvalitet blant lesbiske kvinner og homofile menn [Living Conditions and Life Quality Among Lesbian Women and Gay Men]*. Norsk institutt for forskning om oppvekst, velferd og aldring. Rapport, 1.

Ollendorff Reich, I. (1969), *Wilhelm Reich: A Personal Biography*. London: Elek.

Rado, S. (1940), A critical examination of the concept of bisexuality. *Psychosomatic Medicine*, 2:459-467. Reprinted in *Sexual Inversion: The Multiple Roots of Homosexuality*, ed. J. Marmor. New York: Basic Books, 1965, pp. 175-189.

Rian, Ø. (2001), Mellom straff og fortielse. Homoseksualitet i Norge fra vikingtiden til 1930-årene [Between punishment and silencing. Homosexuality in Norway from the Viking era to the 1930's]. In: *Norsk Homoforskning [Gay Science in Norway]*, eds. M. Brantsæter, T. Eikvam, R. Kjær & K. O. Åmås. Oslo: Universitetsforlaget, pp. 25-56.

Roughton, R. (1995), Overcoming antihomosexual bias: A progress report. *Amer. Psychoanalyst*, 29(4):15-16.

Shidlo, A., Schroeder, M. & Drescher, J. (2001), *Sexual Conversion Therapy: Ethical, Clinical and Research Perspectives*. New York: The Haworth Press, Inc.

Selle, M. (2001), Nei til "behandling"–ja til terapi. En mentalhygienisk veiledning for helsepersonell og pasienter ["Treatment": no–Therapy: yes. Mental health guidelines for health care workers and patients]. In: *Norsk Homoforskning [Gay Science in Norway]*, eds. M. Brantsæter, T. Eikvam, R. Kjær & K. O. Åmås. Oslo: Universitetsforlaget, pp. 238-257.

Stai, A. (1954), *Norsk kultur–og moraldebatt i 1930 årene [The Norwegian Debate on Culture and Morality in the 1930's]*. Oslo: Gyldendal.

Vogt, R. (1905), *Psykiatriens grundtræk I [The Foundations of Psychiatry I]*. Kristiania [Oslo]: Steenske forlag.

Vold, J. E. (2000), *Mørkets sangerske [The Poet of Darkness]*. Oslo: Gyldendal.

Homosexuality in Finland:
The Decline of Psychoanalysis'
Illness Model of Homosexuality

Olli Stålström, PhD
Jussi Nissinen, MSC

SUMMARY. This paper addresses the ways in which Finnish psychiatric textbooks and psychotherapy practices have conceptualized homosexualities since the beginning of the twentieth century. Liberal views of the first decades changed in the 1950s under the influence of the American adaptational (Rado-Bieber) school of psychoanalysis. These later views were reflected in psychiatric textbooks until the 1990s. This paradigm has been criticized since the 1970s by radical psychiatrists and grassroots movements. Changes in American psychiatric textbooks contributed to the change in Finnish textbooks. However, the majority of mental health professionals still feel that their professional training had not given them adequate sources of information about homo/bisexuality and the treatment teams seldom discuss openly the sexual orientation of their clients. *[Article copies available for a fee from The Haworth Document Delivery Service: 1-800-HAWORTH. E-mail address: <getinfo@haworthpressinc. com> Website: <http://www.HaworthPress.com> © 2003 by The Haworth Press, Inc. All rights reserved.]*

Olli Stålström is a sociologist and former lecturer at the University of Kuopio, Finland. He is a board member of STEAM and Co-Editor of FinnQueer web magazine (www.finnqueer.net).

Jussi Nissinen is a psychotherapist and is a board member of STEAM and Co-Editor of FinnQueer web magazine (www.finnqueer.net).

[Haworth co-indexing entry note]: "Homosexuality in Finland: The Decline of Psychoanalysis' Illness Model of Homosexuality." Stålström, Olli, and Jussi Nissinen. Co-published simultaneously in *Journal of Gay & Lesbian Psychotherapy* (The Haworth Medical Press, an imprint of The Haworth Press, Inc.) Vol. 7, No. 1/2, 2003, pp. 75-91; and: *The Mental Health Professions and Homosexuality: International Perspectives* (ed: Vittorio Lingiardi, and Jack Drescher) The Haworth Medical Press, an imprint of The Haworth Press, Inc., 2003, pp. 75-91. Single or multiple copies of this article are available for a fee from The Haworth Document Delivery Service [1-800-HAWORTH, 9:00 a.m. - 5:00 p.m. (EST). E-mail address: getinfo@haworthpressinc. com].

10.1300/J236v07n01_06

KEYWORDS. Adaptational psychiatry, anti-psychiatry, Finnish psychiatry, Finnish psychoanalysis, gay patients, homosexuality, illness model of homosexuality, lesbian patients, mental health professional training, psychiatric textbooks, Rado-Bieber school

THE FIRST WAVE OF PSYCHOANALYSIS IN FINLAND

The arrival of new ideas from the outside into Finland has always been slow. Historian Jan Löfström (1994), in a study of the history of homosexuality in Finland, notes that the acceptance of modern attitudes toward homosexuality in this country did not occur until the middle of the 20th century. Although homosexuality was not a taboo topic, discourse about it was either muted or marginal.[1] There was a slow acceptance of psychoanalysis in Finland as well. For example, the first Finnish-language encyclopedia's 1911 edition (Therman) did not contain any reference to Freud. The entry on homosexuality read, "Homosexual proclivity or sexual attraction to members of the same gender . . . is mainly caused by same-gender persons residing together for long periods (e.g., in monasteries, boarding schools, etc.) or by debauchery" (p. 563).

Juhani Ihanus (1994), a professor of psychology, has written extensively on the history and diffusion of psychoanalytic ideas in Finland. Ihanus believes cultural resistance slowed the arrival of psychoanalytic ideas to Finland in the 1930s. The path-breaking Finnish psychoanalytic pioneer was a medical doctor, Yrjö Kulovesi (1887-1943), who was personally acquainted with Freud and his work. Kulovesi published several articles and books introducing original psychoanalytic ideas into Finland (1933, 1935). Like many continental psychoanalysts of Freud's generation, Kulovesi was a cultured, liberal and tolerant person who valued the ideals of democracy and human rights.[2] In an article in the Finnish medical journal *Duodecim*, Kulovesi (1935) published the first extensive Finnish psychoanalytic article about homosexuality. Kulovesi followed Freud in stating that homosexuality is not an illness, although he nevertheless described homosexuality as a "perversion." Kulovesi argued that most "homosexuals" may never seek psychiatric treatment because they feel no need to be rid of feelings which do not feel like a disorder to them. Kulovesi noted that in some cases, social pressures, discrimination or legal action against "homosexuals" could cause "painful social anxiety." Like Freud, Kulovesi emphasized that homosexuality is not a monolithic entity, but a many-faceted phenomenon. He also warned against using simplified labels, such as "psychopathy" or "degenerate" and against making generalization about "homosexuals" based on studies of patient samples (p. 734). Unfortunately, Kulovesi died prematurely and did not have the time to train followers. Mirroring postfreudian developments in other countries (see Drescher, 1998,

p. 58; Magee and Miller, 1997, p. 61; Lewes, 1988, pp. 24-47), Kulovesi's relatively tolerant approach was followed by a more conservative, psychoanalytic re-reading of the meanings of homosexuality.

CONSERVATIVE, POST-WAR DEVELOPMENTS

In his history of homosexuality in Finland, Löfström (1994) notes that homosexuality as a social identity category began to develop in Finland in the 1950s.[3] In fact, according to Löfström (pp. i-ii), Finnish debates about the social status of homosexuality were almost non-existent until the cold war years. Those were the years when American Senator Joseph McCarthy sought to weed out communists and "homosexuals" from the U.S. Federal Government. In the cold war atmosphere of the early 1950s, these witch-hunts eventually spread to traditionally socially-liberal Scandinavian countries, and resulted in a sharp increase in arrests of gay men in their countries' capitals (Andreasson, 2000).

The symbol of Finnish psychiatric attitudes of that period was a professor of psychiatry at the University of Helsinki, Asser Stenbäck, who was also a priest of the Finnish State Church.[4] As Stenbäck wrote in Swedish, he had an important influence in the whole of Scandinavia where Swedish is the *lingua franca*. As a theologian and psychiatrist, Stenbäck deeply influenced the views on homosexuality of the Finnish state church and of Finnish psychiatry as well during the 1950s and 1960s. He would eventually become one of the main influences responsible for importing the Socarides-Nicolosi (Socarides, 1978; Nicolosi, 1991) views of reparative therapy into Finland and Sweden (Stenbäck 1993).

Stenbäck presented his ethical and scientific arguments in various Christian publications during the 1940s and 1950s. Reflecting a dimension of the political situation in Finland at that time, Stenbäck promoted an ideology of absolute submission to higher authority. For example, because of the invasion by Stalin's Soviet Union in 1939, the Finnish Government had formed a military alliance with Hitler to stop the Soviets. In a letter to a Christian journal, which he entitled, "Ourselves and Greater Finland," Stenbäck exhorted all Finnish citizens to fight for a Greater Finland which would expand it borders to the East ". . . as a tribute to the efforts by Hitler to wipe out the arch-enemy" (Stenbäck, 1941). However, his principle work on sexual ethics was a handbook for teachers, educators, community physicians, theologians and youth counselors which was published by the Committee of Family Education of the Finnish State Church (Stenbäck and Pautola, 1952).

In his role as professor of psychiatry, Stenbäck disassociated himself from Freud's theories of sexuality. Instead, the theoretical framework of Stenbäck's basic text on sexuality paralleled the pathologizing psychoanalytic theories of the Hungarian émigré to the United States, Sandor Rado (1940).[5] Like Rado, Stenbäck believed the biological structure of the genitals is what determines the proper sexual behavior of men and women.[6] According to this perspective, women's genitalia are designed to receive sperm from the man and to give birth to a new human being. According to Stenbäck, this biological fact gives rise to the differences in sexual instincts of men and women: "The male is *active* in seeking his sexual object. The woman is also active but she gives it an expression of the *will to be submissive* to the man" (Stenbäck and Pautola, 1952, p. 43, italicized in original).

In Stenbäck's theory, sexuality can deviate from the heterosexual norm in two ways: masturbation or homosexuality. Onanism, according to Stenbäck, is a widespread disturbance. It is "against Nature" because it does not serve what he believes to be the two basic purposes of sexuality, procreation and child-birth. It is Stenbäck's contention that "modern research" regards masturbation as a symptom of a deep-seated defect or disorder of the total personality (Stenbäck and Pautola, 1952, p. 259).

According to Stenbäck, homosexuality is a "fixation"[7] and a "misdirected sex drive." He also warns that homosexual role modeling and seduction are great dangers: ". . . in many cases, homosexuality has been caused by seduction or other accidental experiences so early that it must be considered a *disease* from the point of view of the individual" (Stenbäck and Pautola, 1952, p. 286, italicized in original). If homosexual seduction feels pleasant, it may become a decisive factor leading toward homosexuality (p. 280). He considers homosexuality to be a "perversion" because the genitals are not used according to the purposes defined by Nature: "Because [homosexuality] does not even fulfill the human need for love, it must be considered to be against Nature" (p. 285).

Stenbäck formulated warnings against the dangers of homosexuality which were later adopted in a 1966 sexual doctrine of the Finnish State Church. For example, Stenbäck claimed that the "homosexual" is morally responsible for the results of expressing his proclivities and therefore has a duty to abstain. The demand for abstention is based on Stenbäck's opinion that homosexuals pose a grave threat to young boys and that their seduction by homosexual men has grave consequences (Stenbäck and Pautola, 1952, p. 288):

> Homosexual proclivities can be contained with the help of the Christian faith and suitable medical help even when they cannot be cured. Although the homosexual is not always responsible for his proclivities, everyone has a duty to refrain from acting it out, in the same way an unmarried person must be celibate. The Bible does not warn about this sin in vain. The increase in homosexuality has always been the expres-

sion of the moral decay of the era. (Evangelical Lutheran Church of Finland, 1966)

Stenbäck further claimed that most "homosexuals" suffer because of their deviation and consequently, most of them would like to overcome their affliction. Stenbäck proposed a plan for the prevention of homosexuality by, for example, deporting homosexuals from their community of residence, as well as the police surveillance of youth clubs, swimming facilities and public toilets (Stenbäck and Pautola, 1952, p. 290). He also recommended castration:

> Many homosexuals, who have been castrated, have even complained that they did not come to be castrated earlier . . . [With the help of early castration] many valuable mental properties that were blocked by homosexuality can bloom . . . The most difficult problem is that some homosexuals, who have lost their hope, do not want to get rid of their habit. (p. 291)

Stenbäck's ideas about homosexuality remained the prevailing psychiatric doctrine on homosexuality in Finland until the 1970s.[8] His religious arguments were later replaced by the Bieberian (Bieber et al., 1962) views imported by another Helsinki professor of psychiatry, the psychoanalyst Kalle Achté. Achté published the first academic textbook of psychiatry in 1971 (Achté, Alanen and Tienari, 1971) in which Irving Bieber was cited as the authority on homosexuality.[9] In his memoirs, Achté (1993) records how important the emerging American psychoanalytic doctrines were for Finnish psychiatry, particularly during the 1950s and early 1960s when the popularity of psychoanalysis was at its highest in the United States. Leading Finnish psychoanalysts and professors of psychiatry of that era, including Achté and others (Tähkä, 1982; Schalin, 1969, 1991; Hägglund, 1981), introduced psychoanalytic theories of homosexuality into this country. Thus, the Rado-Bieber psychoanalytic school and later the Socarides-Nicolosi reparative therapy model became institutionalized for many years in university courses, textbooks, and state church teaching (Stålström, 2001).

Achté reprinted conclusions of the 1962 Bieber study, essentially with only minor revisions, in all the editions of the textbook published between 1971 and 1991. His basic approach follows that of Bieber (Bieber et al., 1962; Bieber, 1967) and defines homosexuality as a "disturbance" and a "fear and inhibition of heterosexual expression" caused by faulty parenting, i.e., a dominating mother and/or a detached father.[10] Achté also claimed that "homosexuals" suffered from the mental disorder of *querulous paranoia*, which he defined as "protesting against real or imagined injustice."[11]

Other prominent, Finnish psychoanalysts who regard homosexuality as psychopathology, in either their texts or teachings, are Veikko Tähkä (1982),

Lars-Olof Schalin (1969, 1991) and Tor-Björn Hägglund (1981). Tähkä, in a widely read handbook on patient-physician relationships, replaced the terms "love," "loved one" and "sexual pleasure" with "disturbance," "patient" and "symptom." Schalin called homosexuality a "disorder" and warned against the seduction of young boys (1991, p. 110). Hägglund also accused "homosexuals" of attempting to molest young boys and compared homosexuality to blinding oneself.[12]

CRITIQUE OF THE ILLNESS MODEL

In Finland, there were four sources of criticism of the illness model of homosexuality. The first came from the growing American empirical research which criticized that model (Kinsey, Pomeroy and Martin, 1948; Kinsey et al., 1953; Ford and Beach, 1951; Hooker, 1957). This research, which was also responsible for the American decision to remove homosexuality from its diagnostic manual, spread to Europe via universities and scientific textbooks.[13] The second source of criticism came from the so-called anti-psychiatric movement of Cooper (1967), Basaglia (1968/1972), R. D. Laing (1971/1973), and Thomas Szasz (1965, 1974). The Norwegian Haugsgjerd (1975/1970) was one of those who introduced anti-psychiatric ideas to Scandinavia. The third source of critique grew out of the remaining influence of the traditional European homosexual emancipation movement, initially inspired by Karl-Heinrich Ulrichs and later embodied in Magnus Hirschfeld's Scientific-Humanitarian Committee (WHK) in the late nineteenth century.[14] The fourth source of critique came from a range of left-wing women's liberation movements from other Scandinavian countries, as well as French existentialism.[15] It should be noted that there was overlap between the four sources insofar as they complemented each other's opposition to traditional ways of thinking about homosexuality.

The Anti-Psychiatry Movement in Finland

A critique of psychiatric violence in general, and of the illness model of homosexuality as well, was introduced to Finland in the early 1960s by an anti-psychiatry movement which was largely inspired by the American psychiatrist and psychoanalyst, Thomas Szasz (1965, 1974). The Finnish pioneers of this movement were two radical medical students, Ilkka Taipale (1966) and Claes Andersson (1968). They organized several debates and panel discussions during the so-called "sex spring" of 1965 and became torchbearers of sexual emancipation. In that year, the Helsinki Student Union newspaper published an issue devoted to the theme of sexuality.[16]

A number of single-issue movements sprang up in the emerging student radicalism: a peace movement, women's liberation, a pedestrian movement and a general anti-authoritarian movement called The November Movement. The sexual radicalism arising largely from anti-authoritarian, critical New Left ideologies was not, however, unconditionally accepting of homosexuality. Two more traditional schools of thought still had a strong hold on people's minds: Marxism and American Psychoanalysis. Some Finnish sexual radicals of the 1960s were only conditionally tolerant of homosexuality. Some adhered to the prevailing Soviet contention that homosexuality, as defined in the Great Soviet Encyclopedia of the 1950s (Vvredenskiy, 1952), was a social pathology of capitalist society. Many left-wing reformers believed that homosexuality would somehow disappear when other social problems of capitalism were overcome. Consequently, although some left-wing radicals of the 1960s half-heartedly supported sexual equality, Moscow-oriented leftists of the 1970s actually opposed sexual equality for gays and lesbians.

A parallel ideological problem among the new left was that to many of its members, orthodox psychoanalysis seemed to offer a set of absolute truths which were above all criticism. Even the radical Claes Andersson, who later became a psychiatrist, author and cabinet minister, was careful not to challenge psychoanalysis in the 1960s. In his preface to Ullerstam's Finnish edition of *Sexual Minorities*, Andersson (1968) demanded the decriminalization of homosexuality and criticized psychiatric stereotypes and dehumanizing psychiatric language. He further describes how Ullerstam had to face a "vicious attack" from the state church and psychoanalysts in Sweden when his book was first published. Nevertheless, Andersson criticized Ullerstam for challenging psychoanalysts, reminding the latter that "psychoanalysts have largely contributed to what we know about the causes of sexual deviations" (p. 7). Andersson argued that "[gays and lesbians] cannot be expected to organize to demand their civil rights." He believed that the best way to help gay people was to enlighten one's own thinking. However, after the gay and lesbian movement had organized in the 1970s, Andersson gave the movement his full support.

Ilkka Taipale is a pioneer of anti-psychiatry and social psychiatry in Finland– a local Thomas Szasz. Taipale also criticized psychiatric terms like "degeneration," "perversion," "psychopathy," "psychosexual infantilism," "neuropathy," etc., which he believes makes it almost impossible to deal "rationally" with the issues surrounding homosexuality. Taipale's arguments draw upon the Kinsey studies, as well as the historical, biological, anthropological and psychiatric studies, which challenged the beliefs that homosexuality would always indicate underlying pathology or that people belonging to sexual minorities would somehow be inferior to others. Taipale further demanded that repressive laws and psychiatric labels be replaced by understanding and acceptance. He criticized a culture that grants sexual satisfaction only to heterosexual individuals, and even then only within marriage. Taipale calls for value-free empirical research and the need for a sexological research institute, which would employ physicians, psychiatrists, biologists, sociologists, anthropologists and historians.

Radical Movements in Finland

International ideas of gay and lesbian liberation began to enter Finland in 1968 from two sources. The first was the traditional European emancipation movement which originated with Magnus Hirschfeld's WHK and continued with the Dutch COC after World War II. A second and later influence was the gay liberation movement in the United States. Nineteen sixty eight was also the peak year of Finnish student radicalism, a time when the Old Student House in Helsinki was occupied and the anti-authoritarian November Movement was founded. The movement's leader, Claes Andersson, criticized the way in which traditional moralism was being transformed into a kind of "humane" neo-intolerance in which the "sexual deviant" now needed "treatment." Small, radical homophile groups emerged alongside the November Movement which published, in 1968 and 1969, two issues of *Homo et societas*, the first homophile magazine in Finland. This magazine introduced radical new visions, from Dutch, Scandinavian and American radical movements, of social equality and integration through confrontation. *Homo et societas* was also the first publication to introduce the comparative studies of Evelyn Hooker in 1968. In the same year, Hooker's (1968) introduction to social scientists in her chapter in the *International Encyclopedia of Social Sciences* further widened the gap between psychoanalysis and the social sciences.

The November Movement provided fertile ground for the development of a general sexual-political movement, SEXPO, and a homophile movement as well (Psyke). The latter was radicalized in 1974 and became the Finnish Organization for Gays and Lesbians (SETA).[17] The emergence of SETA was caused by a general impatience with the cautious politics of the earlier homophile movements; a growing indignation with the antihomosexual attitude of the politically powerful state church of Finland; and the censorship law of 1971 which prevented publication of information about homosexuality.

SETA was also influenced by the American Psychiatric Association's 1973 decision to remove homosexuality from the DSM-II (Bayer, 1981). From its inception, SETA strongly criticized psychoanalysis' illness label of homosexuality.[18] SETA took the position that while homosexuality is not a disorder, discrimination and societal pressure against gay people could lead to their developing mental problems and suicidal thoughts–unless proper help was made available. It urged a total revision of what was written about homosexuality in psychiatric and medical textbooks, in the field of mental health education, and suicide prevention. SETA further demanded that homosexuality be deleted from the national classification of disease.

1981: THE FINNISH DECLASSIFICATION OF HOMOSEXUALITY

The momentum to formally delete homosexuality from the World Health Organization (WHO) classification used in Finland began in the late 1970s. The Finnish gay rights movement was assisted by Michael W. Ross, a New Zealand psychiatrist who did post-graduate studies and research at both the Universities of Helsinki and Stockholm at that time (see Ross, Paulsen and Stålström, 1988). With his assistance, Finnish medical authorities were made aware of earlier decisions to declassify homosexuality as a mental disorder in Australia (1973), the United States (1973), Norway (1978) and Sweden (1978). In 1978, Ross even gave a guest lecture at Achté's (see above) psychiatric hospital, informing his Finnish colleagues about new research in psychiatry.[19] He also gave interviews on the subject in the Finnish daily press.

SETA repeatedly requested of the Finnish Board of Health to bring its classification system into line with other Western countries and to remove the diagnostic category of *Anomaliae sexuales* (302.00). SETA argued that the diagnosis had a wider significance beyond its usage as a code for medical documents, noting it was used to stigmatize gays and lesbians–even in high school textbooks (SETA, 1979). The Finnish Board of Health's initial response paralleled the 1973 APA decision to replace homosexuality per se with ego-dystonic homosexuality (Bayer, 1987). The Board recommended that the diagnostic labels in group 302 should not be used *unless the patient her/himself has come to treatment for problems in this diagnostic category* (National Board of Health, 1980, emphasis added).

This compromise was unacceptable to SETA and to many Finnish psychiatrists as well; they demanded the unconditional deletion of the diagnostic category. After a heated public debate, and citing precedents in other Nordic countries, the Finnish National Board of Health ruled that the diagnostic codes referring to "sexual anomalies" would no longer be used in Finland (National Board of Health, 1981).

PSYCHIATRIC TEXTBOOKS

From 1971 to 1991, each edition of Achté's textbook, *Psykiatria*, continued to pathologize homosexuality from a Bieberian perspective. Even after the diagnostic classification of homosexuality was deleted from the Finnish diagnostic classification in 1981, Achté refused to change the pathological labeling of homosexuality. Even the 1992 formal demand by the Student Union of the University of Helsinki that the books be updated or be withdrawn had no effect. The textbook was never updated.[20]

Traditionally, American textbooks are highly esteemed in Scandinavia. In a 1996 televised retirement interview, Achté said the books he valued most were the Bible and Kaplan and Sadock's *Comprehensive Textbook of Psychiatry*. It seems the pathological labeling of homosexuality in Finland could not end before the American source itself changed. Consequently, it was an event of international significance when Terry Stein (2000) wrote a chapter in the 7th edition of Kaplan and Sadock which discarded the pathologizing labels and psychoanalytic stereotypes of previous editions (Gadpaille, 1995). In fact, a completely new Finnish psychiatric textbook, *Psykiatria*, was published by a new generation of psychiatrists (see Heikkinen, 1999). This textbook closely follows the American DSM-IV classification in which homosexuality is not mentioned. It also makes it clear that homosexuality is no longer considered a clinical entity and rebuts some of the most widespread psychoanalytic theories that claim it is.

There is a startling episode in the Finnish textbook debate which involved one of this paper's authors (Stålström). In 1997, Stålström published his doctoral dissertation on the history and removal of the diagnostic label of homosexuality in the Unites States and Finland: *The End of the Sickness Label of Homosexuality*. In his dissertation, Stålström criticized the work of a Finnish psychiatrist, Kaija Eerola (1996). One of his criticisms was that Eerola had defined homosexuality in terms of deviance and disturbance and referred to this as the "prevailing view" in Finland on the subject. She subsequently sued Stålström for libel. After police interrogations, the public prosecutor brought libel charges against Stålström and his publisher, Helsinki University Press. The prosecutor's office also demanded the wholesale confiscation of all published copies of the dissertation as well as a financial compensation of 50,000 Euros[21] to Eerola.

These unprecedented court proceedings drew international attention. Concerned about Finland's international reputation, an umbrella organization representing all Finnish publishers retained an internationally known human rights lawyer and Member of European Parliament, Matti Wuori, for the defense. Many expert witness, from both Finland and abroad, either testified or submitted written statements refuting the scientific claims of Eerola's chapter.[22] The Municipal Court of Tampere issued its verdict on December 18, 1999 and found Stålström not guilty of libel and all demands for compensation were denied.[23]

MENTAL HEALTH PROFESSIONAL ATTITUDES
TOWARD GLB PATIENTS

In the last decade, there appears to be a paradigm shift taking place in relation to homo/bisexuality in Finnish health care. Nevertheless, there is little open dialogue about the needs of GLB patients. There are several studies about the attitudes of Finnish mental health professionals toward gay, lesbian and bisexual patients/clients. Valtanen (1990) studied attitudes of physicians, psychotherapists, and nurses working in mental health care outpatient units toward homosexual patients. In all three professional categories, more than one half of those surveyed felt that their professional training had not given them adequate sources of information about homo/bisexuality. Instead, the respondents stated they found newspaper articles, radio and television programs and their own clients to be the best sources of information.

There is some new empirical data regarding workers in the health care field and homo- and bisexuality in Finland. Nissinen (1995) measured the attitudes of and knowledge about homo/bisexuality among physicians, therapists, social workers, nurses and other staff (N = 200) working in substance abuse outpatient and inpatient service units. According to these studies, 7-10% of respondents had homophobic reactions to homosexuality on the Hudson and Rickerts scale (Hudson & Rickerts, 1980). Nissinen also found that treatment teams did not openly discuss the sexuality of their homo/bisexual clients. This lack of discussion could explain how one therapist estimated that about 10% of his clients had been homo/bisexual, whereas another therapist, practicing the same number of years on the same treatment team, believed he had never encountered a single lesbian, gay or bisexual client. One therapist in a unit might refer a lesbian/gay/bisexual client to reparative therapy, whereas another one might work using a gay-affirmative approach. The great majority of therapists, however, totally ignore the issue of a patient's sexual orientation.

Therapists reported uncertainty about how to discuss homosexuality in an open way. Some feared heterosexist/homophobic attitudes of colleagues based upon comments they made. Respondents also had little understanding of gay identity formation. Some thought of homo/bisexuality solely as a personal identity but did not know much about the value of social identification and peer groups. In addition, homo/bisexual professionals could be accepted on an individual basis as colleagues, but the respondents did not consider it appropriate for gay, lesbian and bisexual professionals to form networks.

TRAINING OF PSYCHOTHERAPISTS

At the present time in Finland, scarce attention is paid to homo/bisexuality in the training of health care professionals. An exception can be found in the paraprofessional and intermediate level institutes (Polytechnics) which train ancillary health care personnel, including nurses. These programs have actively included courses on sexuality and diversity in their training program which they developed with the assistance of gay and lesbian organizations

(SETA). In contrast, university-level teaching (physicians, psychologists, social workers) and professional education (psychotherapy training, family therapy training) either totally ignore health care issues regarding sexual minorities or address them superficially.

In 1996, the Organization for Lesbian, Gay and Bisexual Professionals within Health Care and Social Work (STEAM) was founded. Its aim is to serve as a network providing support and information and develop training and job supervision for professionals. As part of its mission, in early 2001 STEAM sent a questionnaire to about 20 organizations which organize psychotherapy training. One of the original goals of the questionnaire was to gather information for this article. It asked the training organizations how they dealt with a client's homo/bisexuality in their training programs. The questionnaire also asked them whether they would be interested in cooperating with STEAM in the development of GLB-sensitive training. Only one organization bothered to reply to the questionnaire and its answers were so superficial that no useful data was provided.

In the absence of more systematically gathered information, there is only anecdotal data to report. In the psychotherapy training and job supervision experience of one author (Jussi Nissinen), homo/bisexuality is seldom openly discussed. When it is, homosexuality is often defined as a problem to be explained or a form of disturbance/arrested development. There is little attention paid to the kinds of problems that homo/bisexual clients face in interactions with their heterosexist social environments. In Nissinen's training in family therapy, senior teachers express the belief that same-gendered partnerships do not form a good basis for the emotional growth of children. Clearly, more work is needed in this area. In fact, as open gay and lesbian mental health professionals have increasingly entered the field in the 1990s (Lehtonen, Nissinen and Socada, 1997), they have begun to have an impact on the training and practice of psychotherapy.

NOTES

1. Löfström believes this is because gender roles of men and women in Finland were not considered mutually exclusive categories.

2. In his biography of Kulovesi, Ihanus tells how Kulovesi tried to oppose the rising right-wing conservative and nationalist movement, which in the 1930s extended its influence from Germany to Finland as well.

3. This change was caused, in Löfström's analysis, by emerging urbanization, industrialization, the strengthening position of the Finnish middle class, the rise of a bureaucratic society and medical profession, and the challenges posed by changing gender roles.

4. Stenbäck, ordained as a priest in 1935, worked as a Chaplain in the Finnish State Church from 1935 to 1947. He was also a professor of psychiatry at the universities of Turku and Helsinki from 1964 to 1976.

5. Rado's work has been noted by some authors as a decisive antihomosexual turning point in psychoanalytic theorizing about homosexuality (see Bayer, 1987; Lewes 1988; Drescher 1998).

6. Editor's Note: As Rado put it, "The male-female sexual pattern is dictated by anatomy" (Rado, S. 1969), *Adaptational Psychodynamics: Motivation and Control*. New York: Science House, p. 212).

7. Editor's Note: This is consistent with one of Freud's theories of homosexuality, particularly as described in his account of Leonardo da Vinci. See Freud, S. (1910), Leonardo da Vinci and a memory of his childhood. *Standard Edition*, 11:59-138. London: Hogarth Press, 1957.

8. After retiring from psychiatry, Stenbäck continued his opposition to homosexuality as a Christian Member of the Finnish Parliament. Stenbäck introduced the Nicolosi-Socarides version of reparative therapy to Scandinavia in the 1990s with a booklet, in Swedish, distributed by the Swedish organization, Save the Family. The booklet was distributed to all Members of the Swedish Parliament. It was then immediately translated into Finnish (Stenbäck, 1993).

9. Achté included his friend and colleague Asser Stenbäck on the editorial board of the Finnish textbook of psychiatry until 1981.

10. A content analysis by Stålström (1977) indicates that Achté claims a number of mental disorders and problems associated with homosexuality.

11. This became a psychoanalytic, rhetorical mechanism against those gays and lesbians who protested against discrimination. Stålström (1980) has compared this type of psychiatric labeling with the silencing of dissidents in the former Soviet Union. [Editor's Note: The American version of this approach was first put forward in the 1950s by Edmund Bergler, a psychiatrist and psychoanalyst who referred to his homosexual patients as "injustice collectors." See Bergler, E. (1956), *Homosexuality: Disease or Way of Life*. New York: Hill & Wang. This concept was later resuscitated by Nicolosi (1991).]

12. For a more detailed analysis see Stålström, 1997, pp. 237-248.

13. Kinsey's *Sexual Behavior in the Human Female* was translated into Finnish one year after its American publication. Evelyn Hooker's studies entered the universities mainly through the social sciences and scientific handbooks. As a result, these newer ideas had their first impact felt in the social sciences, and professors of the social sciences have traditionally been important allies of the gay and lesbian movement in Finland.

14. Editor's Note: See Lauritsen, J. & Thorstad, D. (1974), *The Early Homosexual Rights Movement (1864-1935)*. New York: Times Change Press.

15. Simone de Beauvoir (1949/1980) and Jean-Paul Sartre (1943/1969) both had an influence that reached Scandinavia through various women's consciousness-raising groups.

16. The debates were inspired by the Swedish reformer, Lars Ullerstam, whose 1964 book was translated into English translated as *The Erotic Minorities* and into

Finnish in 1968. Ullerstam's book was a sharp critique of the psychiatric culture which pathologized all non-procreative sexuality.

17. Tarja Halonen, a human rights lawyer, was a founding member of SEXPO, became the chairwoman of SETA in 1980 and eventually the President of Finland in 2000.

18. One of the first articles criticizing the psychoanalytic label of homosexuality was published by Stålström (1975). It was mainly a critique of the psychoanalytic theory of homosexuality based on the empirical findings of Hooker and the social critique of Ullerstam, Sartre and Szasz.

19. Achté, however, dismissed these views and stated that "Irving Bieber is my authority and will remain my authority" (quoted in Stålström, 1997, p. 229).

20. Even after retirement, professor Achté continues the psychoanalytic tradition of indiscriminately applying psychoanalytic labels and descriptions to homosexual and other artists. In his book about the gay Finnish poet, Uuno Kailas, Achté (2001, p. 15) reviews literary studies of almost 50 authors and poets and concludes that all of them, with the exception of Guy de Maupassant, suffered from serious psychiatric disorders. The following authors are listed as psychiatrically disturbed: Brecht, Camus, Dostoyevsky, Faulkner, Gide, Gogol, Hemingway, Hesse, Ibsen, Joyce, Kafka, Kipling, Proust, Sartre, Strindberg, Tolstoy, Wells, Wilde, Zola.

21. Almost $50,000 US.

22. These included a Finnish psychiatrist Martti Heikkinen (1999); Professor Ilkka Niiniluoto, Vice Rector of the University of Helsinki; Michael W. Ross of the University of Texas; Ellen Mercer of the American Psychiatric Association's Office of International Affairs; Jack Drescher, Chair of the APA's Committee on Gay, Lesbian and Bisexual Issues; and Ralph Roughton, speaking for the American Psychoanalytic Association.

23. The psychiatric expert of Weilin + Göös did not appeal the court's decision. The court proceedings had already generated innumerable articles in the national press. The scientific community in Finland and abroad felt the verdict as a relief. Ross (forthcoming) wrote an analysis of the court proceedings, based on his interviews with the key Finnish actors in the case and the police investigation record.

REFERENCES

Achté, K., Alanen, Y. O. & Tienari, P. (1971), *Seksuaalitoiminnan häiriöt ja seksuaaliset poikkeamat* [Disturbances and deviations of sexual activities]. In: *Psykiatria [Psychiatry]*, eds. K. Achté, Y. O. Alanen, & P. Tienari. First edition. Porvoo: WSOY, pp. 638-656.

Achté, K. (1993), *Lääkärikoulussa Paasikiven aikaan [In Medical School in the Time of President Paasikivi]*. Vaasa: Recallmed.

Achté, K. (2001), *Uuno Kailas. Runoilija psykiatrin silmin (Uuno Kailas: A Poet Seen Through the Eyes of a Psychiatrist)*. Helsinki: Helsinki University Press.

Andersson, C. (1968), *Johdanto* [Introduction]. In: *Sukupuoliset vähemmistöt [Sexual Minorities]*, ed. L. Ullerstam. Helsinki: Tammi, pp. 5-8.

Andreasson, M., ed. (2000), *Homo I folkhemmet. Homo-och bisexuella i Sverige 1950-2000* [*Homo in the Peoples' Home: Homo/Bisexuality in Sweden*, 1950-2000]. Göteborg: Anamma.

Basaglia, F. (1968), *Kumous laitosmaailmassa* [*Negated Institutions*]. Translated by Pirkko Peltonen. Helsinki: Tammi, 1972.

Bayer, R. (1987), *Homosexuality and American Psychiatry: The Politics of Diagnosis.* Second Edition. New York: Basic Books.

Bieber, I., Dain, H., Dince, P., Drellich, M., Grand, H., Gundlach, R., Kremer, M., Rifkin, A., Wilbur, C. & Bieber T. (1962), *Homosexuality: A Psychoanalytic Study.* New York: Basic Books.

Bieber, I. (1967), Sexual deviations. In: *Comprehensive Textbook of Psychiatry*, eds. A. M. Freedman & H. I. Kaplan. First edition. Baltimore, MD: William & Wilkins, pp. 959-976.

Cooper, D. (1967), *Psychiatry and Anti-Psychiatry.* London: Tavistock.

de Beauvoir, S. (1949), *Toinen sukupuoli* [*The Second Sex*]. Translated by Annikki Suni. Helsinki: Kirjayhtymä, 1980.

Drescher, J. (1998), *Psychoanalytic Therapy and the Gay Man.* Hillsdale, NJ: The Analytic Press.

Evangelical Lutheran Church of Finland (1966), *Ajankohtainen asia* [*A Topical Issue*]. Statement of the Bishops: Helsinki.

Eerola, K. (1996), *Seksuaaliset vähemmistöt* [Sexual minorities]. In: *Suomalainen lääkärikeskus* [*Finnish Medical Center*] ed. M. Huttunen. Second, revised edition, Volume 2. Porvoo: Weilin + Göös, pp. 395-401.

Ford, C. & Beach, F. (1951), *Patterns of Sexual Behavior.* New York: Harper.

Gadpaille, W. J. (1995), Homosexuality and homosexual activity. In: *Comprehensive Textbook of Psychiatry, Volume 2*, eds. H. I. Kaplan & B. Sadock. Sixth edition. Baltimore, MD: William & Wilkins, pp. 1321-1333.

Hägglund, T.-B. (1981), *Seksuaalinen poikkeavuus* [Sexual deviation]. *Kaleva*, November 14.

Haugsgjerd, S. (1975/1970), *Psykiatria ja yhteiskunta* [*Psychiatry and Society*]. Translated by Eira Stenberg. Tapiola: Weilin + Göös.

Heikkinen, M. (1999), *Seksuaalihäiriöt* [Sexual disturbances]. In: *Psykiatria* [*Psychiatry*], eds. J. Lönnqvist, M. Heikkinen, M. Henriksson, M. Marttunen & T. Partonen. Helsinki: Duodecim, pp. 322-342.

Hooker, E. (1957), The adjustment of the male overt homosexual. *J. Proj. Tech*, 21:18-31.

Hooker, E. (1968), Homosexuality. In: *International Encyclopedia of the Social Sciences*, ed. D. L. Sills. New York: Macmillan, pp. 222-233.

Hudson, W. W. & Ricketts, W. A. (1980), A strategy for measurement of homophobia. *J. Homosex.*, 5(4):357-372.

Ihanus, J. (1994), *Vietit vai henki. Psykoanalyysin varhaisvaiheet Suomessa* [*Instinct or Spirit: Early Stages of Psychoanalysis in Finland*]. Helsinki: Helsinki University Press.

Kinsey, A., Pomeroy, W. & Martin, C. (1948), *Sexual Behavior in the Human Male.* Philadelphia, PA: Saunders.

Kinsey, A., Pomeroy, W., Martin, C. & Gebhard, P. (1953), *Sexual Behavior in the Human Female*. Philadelphia, PA: Saunders.

Kulovesi, Y. (1933), *Psykoanalyysi [Psychoanalysis]*. Helsinki: Otava.

Kulovesi, Y. (1935), *Perversiteettien psyykillisestä rakenteesta* [On the psychological structure of perversions]. *Duodecim*, 51:734-739.

Laing, R. D. (1971), *Perhesuhteiden politiikka [The Politics of the Family]*. Translated by Elina Hytönen. Helsinki: Otava, 1973.

Lehtonen, J., Nissinen, J. & Socada, M. (1997), *Hetero-olettamuksesta moninaisuuteen* [*From Hetero Assumption to Diversity*]. Helsinki: Edita.

Lewes, K. (1988), *The Psychoanalytic Theory of Male Homosexuality*. New York: Simon and Schuster. Reissued as *Psychoanalysis and Male Homosexuality* (1995), Northvale, NJ: Aronson.

Löfström, J. (1994), The Social Construction of Homosexuality in Finnish Society: From the Late Nineteenth Century to the 1950s. Unpublished Ph.D. thesis, University of Essex, Department of Sociology.

Magee, M. & Miller, D. (1997), *Lesbian Lives: Psychoanalytic Narratives Old and New*. Hillsdale, NJ: The Analytic Press.

National Board of Health (1980), Circular Letter No. 1734, Dno 6680/02/80, *Correction to the Classification of Disorders and Causes of Death* (ratified on January 1, 1969). Helsinki, November 17.

National Board of Health (1981), Circular Letter No. 1754, Dno 4043/02/81, *Deletion of the diagnostic label of homosexuality. Correction to the Classification of Disorders and Cause of Death* (ratified on January 1, 1969). Helsinki, June 26.

Nicolosi, J. (1991), *Reparative Therapy of Male Homosexuality: A New Clinical Approach*. Northvale, NJ: Aronson.

Nissinen, J. (1995), *Homo-ja biseksuaalisuuden huomioonottaminen päihdehuollossa* [*Taking Homo/Bisexuality into Account in Substance Abuse Counseling*]. MSc thesis, University of Helsinki, Department of Social Psychology.

Rado, S. (1940), A critical examination of the concept of bisexuality. *Psychosomatic Medicine*, 2:459-467. Reprinted in *Sexual Inversion: The Multiple Roots of Homosexuality*, ed. J. Marmor. New York: Basic Books, 1965, pp. 175-189.

Ross, M. W., Paulsen, J. A. & Stålström, O. W. (1988), Homosexuality and mental health: A cross-cultural review. In: *The Treatment of Homosexuals with Mental Health Disorders*, ed. M. Ross. New York: Harrington Park Press.

Ross, M. W. (forthcoming), The last book-burning trial of the 20th century: The Stålström case and the sickness label of homosexuality. *J. Gay & Lesb. Psychother.*

Sartre, J. P. (1943), *Being and Nothingness*. London: Methuen, 1969.

Schalin, L.-O. (1969), *Psykoanalyysin näkemys yksilön kehityksestä* (Psychoanalytic view of individual development). In: *Psykologian sovelluksia [Applications of Psychology]*, ed. M. Takala. Helsinki: Weilin + Göös.

Schalin, L.-O. (1991), *Perheen ihmissuhteista* [*On Human Relationships in the Family*]. Helsinki: Helsinki University Press.

SETA (1979), Memorandum to the National Board of Health, October 29.

Socarides, C. (1978), *Homosexuality*. New York: Jason Aronson.

Stålström, O. (1975), *Ennakkoluulot, yhteiskunnan kehityshäiriö* [Prejudice, a developmental disturbance of society]. *SETA* [Magazine of the Gay and Lesbian Organization of Finland], 1:8.

Stålström, O. (1977), *Homoseksuaalisuus–sairautta vai rakkautta* [Homosexuality: Disorder or love). *Medisiinari*, 6:18-24.

Stålström, O. (1980), Querulous paranoia: Diagnosis and dissent. *Australian & New Zealand J. Psychiatry*, 14:145-150.

Stålström, O. (1997), *Homoseksuaalisuuden sairausleiman loppu* [*The End of the Sickness Label of Homosexuality*]. PhD dissertation. Helsinki: Gaudeamus.

Stålström, O. (2001), *Asser Stenbäck, Kalle Achté ja Lars-Olof Schalin–eheytysliikeen esi-isiä Suomessa* [*The founding fathers of the Finnish reparative therapy movement: Asser Stenbäck, Kalle Achté and Lars-Olof Schalin*]. *Finnqueer Web Magazine*, section *Eheytys* [Reparative therapy], February 7, http://www.finnqueer.net/juttu.cgi?s=40_10_1.

Stein, T. (2000), Homosexuality and homosexual behavior. In: *Comprehensive Textbook of Psychiatry*, Volume 2, eds. B. Sadock & V. Sadock. Seventh edition. Baltimore, MD: William & Wilkins, pp. 1608-1631.

Stenbäck, A. (1941), *Vi och Stor-Finland* [Ourselves and Greater Finland]. *Ad Lucem*, 5:36 (October).

Stenbäck, A. & Pautola, L. (1952), *Lapsuus-ja nuoruusiän sukupuolinen kehitys ja kasvatus* [*Sexual Development and Upbringing in Childhood and Adolescence*]. Helsinki: Otava.

Stenbäck, A. (1993), *Mitä homoseksuaalisuus on? [What is Homosexuality?*]. Hämeenlinna: SLEY kirjat.

Szasz, T. (1965), Legal and moral aspects of homosexuality. In: *Sexual Inversion: The Multiple Roots of Homosexuality*, ed. J. Marmor. New York: Basic Books, pp. 124-139.

Szasz, T. (1974), *The Myth of Mental Illness: Foundations of a Theory of Personal Conduct*, Revised Edition. New York: Harper & Row.

Taipale, I., ed. (1966), *Sukupuoleton Suomi (Sexless Finland)*. Helsinki: Tammi.

Tähkä, V. (1982), *Psykoterapian perusteet psykoanalyyttisen terapian pohjalta [Basics of Psychotherapy Based on Psychoanalytic Theory*]. Porvoo: WSOY.

Therman, E. (1911), *Homoseksuaalisuus* [Homosexuality]. In: *Tietosanakirja [Encyclopedia*], ed. Y. Wickman, Helsinki: Otava, p. 563.

Ullerstam, L. (1968), *Sukupuoliset vähemmistöt* [*Sexual Minorities*]. Translated by Esko Kärnä. Helsinki: Tammi.

Valtanen, K. (1990), *Mielenterveyspalvelu ja homoseksuaalinen asiakas* [*Mental Health Services and the Homosexual Patient*]. University of Oulu. Department of Public Health.

Vvredenskiy, B. A., ed. (1952), *Gomoseksualism* [Homosexuality]. In: *Bol´shaya Sovetskaya Entsiklopedia (Great Soviet Encyclopedia)*. Moscow: Bol´shaya Sovetskaya Entsiklopedia, p. 35.

Happy Italy?
The Mediterranean Experience
of Homosexuality, Psychoanalysis,
and the Mental Health Professions

Paola Capozzi, MD
Vittorio Lingiardi, MD

SUMMARY. The authors outline the history of the relationship between Italian psychoanalytic and psychiatric institutions and homosexuality. In a "don't ask-don't tell" climate, this history evolved between post-war Italy's ideological polarization between Catholicism and post-war Marxism as well as between two different "local cultures": Middle-European and Mediterranean. In a review of the Italian psychoanalytic,

Paola Capozzi is Psychiatrist and Psychoanalyst affiliated with the Società Psicoanalitica Italiana (SPI), the International Psychoanalytic Association (IPA), and the International Association for Relational Psychoanalysis and Psychotherapy (IARPP). She is in private practice in Milan, Italy.

Vittorio Lingiardi is Professor, Faculty of Psychology, University of Rome "La Sapienza." He is Psychiatrist and Psychoanalyst affiliated with the Centro Italiano di Psicologia Analitica (CIPA), the International Association for Analytical Psychology (IAAP), and the International Association for Relational Psychoanalysis and Psychotherapy (IARPP). He is in private practice in Milan, Italy.

Address correspondence to: Paola Capozzi, via Ramazzini, 7. 20129, Milan, Italy (E-mail: paolacapozzi@tiscalinet.it) or Vittorio Lingiardi, via San Vito, 26. 20123, Milan, Italy (E-mail: taovit@micronet.it).

The authors wish to thank Franco De Masi and Luca Formenton for their support while writing this paper.

[Haworth co-indexing entry note]: "Happy Italy? The Mediterranean Experience of Homosexuality, Psychoanalysis, and the Mental Health Professions." Capozzi, Paola, and Vittorio Lingiardi. Co-published simultaneously in *Journal of Gay & Lesbian Psychotherapy* (The Haworth Medical Press, an imprint of The Haworth Press, Inc.) Vol. 7, No. 1/2, 2003, pp. 93-116; and: *The Mental Health Professions and Homosexuality: International Perspectives* (ed: Vittorio Lingiardi, and Jack Drescher) The Haworth Medical Press, an imprint of The Haworth Press, Inc., 2003, pp. 93-116. Single or multiple copies of this article are available for a fee from The Haworth Document Delivery Service [1-800-HAWORTH, 9:00 a.m. - 5:00 p.m. (EST). E-mail address: getinfo@haworthpressinc.com].

10.1300/J236v07n01_07

psychological and psychiatric literature from 1930 to the present, there is a dearth of articles dealing with homosexuality. In the articles that do exist, most link homosexuality with psychopathology or developmental arrests. There is no discussion of the concept of internalized homophobia in the Italian literature. The authors present some early, empirical research in which they assess attitudes toward homosexuality among members of Italian psychoanalytic institutions, both Freudian and Jungian. Preliminary data indicates a greater antihomosexual bias in Freudian institutes. The authors conclude that in the last ten years the cultural climate and the clinical attitude have changed and that the Italian mental health community is beginning to come to terms with its own antihomosexual biases. *[Article copies available for a fee from The Haworth Document Delivery Service: 1-800-HAWORTH. E-mail address: <getinfo@haworthpressinc. com> Website: <http://www.HaworthPress.com> © 2003 by The Haworth Press, Inc. All rights reserved.]*

KEYWORDS. Analytical psychology, discrimination, "don't ask, don't tell," homophobia, homosexuality, Italian psychoanalysis, Italian psychiatry, psychoanalytic training, theories of homosexuality

In order to understand the attitude of Italian psychoanalysts and psychiatrists with respect to homosexuality, one must bear in mind two double-sided trademarks of Italian culture: (1) Catholicism and post-war Marxism, and (2) a Mediterranean identity but also a Middle-European one. Moreover, social relationships in Italy have always been characterized by the personal and political practice of "don't ask-don't tell." In spite of the Pope's presence, Italy was one of the first European countries to decriminalize homosexuality[1] and one could reasonably say that Italy is a gay-friendly country. In the days of the Grand Tour, Italy was considered to be a paradise for gay intellectuals and travellers from Northern Europe (Aldrich, 1993). The following is Roger Peyrefitte's testimony (1949, p. 155), taken from an account of the life of Baron von Gloeden:

Happy Italy! Happy Sicily! There are imbeciles here, too, like anywhere else, who would be pleased to do some harm; but rarely do they have the opportunity. Because in considering these matters, there is the question of intelligence, and the Italian population, being the most intelligent on earth, considers gays in the most indulgent way, well aware of the fact, furthermore, that in the whole course of its history, the most glorious names followed the Greek tradition, that in vain they've tried to render infamous. Maybe it is not incompatible with infamy, but then nor is it with glory. (our translation)

In any event, Freud (1935), citing Leonardo da Vinci and Michelangelo in his famous *Letter to an American Mother*, said things that were not dissimilar: "Homosexuality is assuredly no advantage, but it is nothing to be ashamed of, no vice, no degradation. . ."

THE BIRTH OF THE PSYCHOANALYTIC MOVEMENT IN ITALY

One can speak of Italian psychoanalysis as a movement only after the last world war. Before that time, in fact, psychoanalysis in Italy was approached only by individuals from the academic world, such as Cesare Musatti.[2] Between the two world wars, the only Italian psychoanalyst of international renown was Edoardo Weiss. A Triestine forced to emigrate to the United States at the outbreak of Fascism, Weiss had been analyzed by Paul Federn in Vienna and was a personal acquaintance of Freud. Weiss analyzed Umberto Saba, one of the most important of Italian poets and the author of an unfinished and posthumously published novel, *Ernesto*. A controversial and tormented homosexual, although married to the beloved Lina, Saba, at the age of 46, began a therapeutic relationship with Weiss during the first months of 1929.[3] In a letter dated September 13, 1929, Saba confidentially informs Giacomo Debenedetti that he had rather reluctantly undergone treatment with Weiss due to a crisis which had made him not only think of suicide, but to actually prepare for it. In this letter Saba writes:

> For many years now I have been battling with the idea of whether to go in for this therapy or not: but there were too many resistances and oppositions from the outside . . . One of the main ones . . . was a false interpretation of one of Freud's passages, from which I had deducted that my case was incurable.[4] But desperation forced me into trying. (quoted in Pavanello Accerboni, 1984, p. 552)

Saba, however, goes on to say:

> I'm better, and better in a new way; in a way that has nothing to do with my previous improvements: something in my soul has changed, changed forever . . . You should understand that at the root of my illness was the lack of a father. (quoted in Marcovecchio, 1983, p. 180)

However, in another letter written to the poet Vittorio Sereni in 1952, Saba, after the passing of many years, recalls his experience with Weiss:

> In reality, rather than *heal*, I personally understood many more things about the human soul, that before I was not only in the dark about but

knew nothing of. The worst thing about my childhood was the absence of a father (either good or bad), and Doctor Weiss filled this role, up to a point, filled this lack. Anyway, by the time he left, I was much better, and he was able to say to my wife: *Your husband is not cured but is much better.* (in Lavagetto, 1981, p. 410)

In some ways, the official account of the Weiss-Saba case exemplifies both the beginnings of psychoanalysis in Italy, and at the same time contains all the ingredients that make up the "Italian" relationship between psychoanalysis and homosexuality that remained unaltered right up to the 1990s: deafening silence and affectionate welcome. It cannot be ignored, for example, that in an article published by *Rivista di Psicoanalisi* (Pavanello Accerboni, 1984) entitled "Umberto Saba's 'Personal Myth' between Poetry and Psychoanalysis," there is no mention of the poet's homosexuality. This is a rather glaring omission insofar as two years earlier, Savo Spaçal (1982) had written an article about Edoardo Weiss's psychoanalytic contribution in the same journal and one of the cases reported was, without any doubt, that of Weiss' treatment of Saba. While the relationship between Weiss and Saba appeared to be both respectful and affectionate, it is likely there was collusion between them in favor of a reparative therapy *ante litteram* ("your husband is not cured but is much better"). Saba, unsettled about an anticipated meeting with Weiss many years after the treatment, wrote:

Today I await Doctor Weiss, who has come to Trieste for a few days. But what will I say to him after so many years? The only thing that would be suitable is Essenin's verse, written in a letter to his mother: 'Don't meddle with that which has not worked out.' (quoted in Pavanello Accerboni, 1984, p. 547)

Italy's psychoanalytic movement began to take shape after the fall of Fascism in 1945, spearheaded by a few socialist intellectuals including Musatti in Milan and Emilio Servadio and Nicola Perrotti in Rome. In those days, advocating for psychoanalysis was a difficult and radically alternative path, one that did not have the backing of either academia or medical institutions. On the contrary, Italian psychiatrists of that time were mostly organicists who devalued psychoanalysis. Paradigmatically, Ugo Cerletti, the inventor of electroconvulsive therapy, was Italian. In addition, psychoanalysis was fought, if not actually demonized, by Italy's Catholic culture. Finally, even after the fall of Fascism, there continued to prevail a strong anti-psychoanalytic prejudice among the Italian left. From the Marxist, positivistic point of view, psychoanalysis was looked upon with suspicion. Nevertheless the Italian psychoanalytic movement managed to take root.

THE JUNGIANS IN ITALY

One of the authors of this paper (Lingiardi) was trained as a Jungian analyst. To sum up the history of analytical psychology in Italy (Kirsch, 2000), one must remember that a stable group of Jungian analysts was only formed at the end of the 1950s through the efforts of a German psychiatrist, Ernst Bernhard and his pupil Hélène Erba Tissot. In 1961, the Italian Association of Analytical Psychology (AIPA) was founded and in 1966 the Italian Centre of Analytical Psychology (CIPA). Both groups belong to the International Association for Analytical Psychology (IAAP). In Italy, post-Jungian psychology has developed two principal branches: (a) a phenomenological-hermeneutic approach engaged in dialogue with psychoanalysis and which has abandoned Jung's "esotericism"; and (b) an archetypal approach characterized, among other things by the diffusion in Italy of the ideas of James Hillman (1972, 1991) and with ties to the Jung Institute in Zurich.

Jungian Italian publishers (RED Edizioni, Vivarium) pay attention to foreign contributions on homosexuality, and have translated books by the Swiss Paul Schellenbaum (1991) and the American Christine Downing (1991). A review of the Italian Jungian literature indicates, with the exception of a few works (Carotenuto, 1982; Lingiardi, 1995; Lucchini, 1997), a dearth of papers on homosexuality. One could say that the post-Jungian canon confirms Jung's lack of interest in sexual behaviors. Other post-Jungian contributions include Carotenuto's (1985) essay on Pier Paolo Pasolini, *The Fall of Conscience*, and Lingiardi's book (1997) *Men in Love: Male Homosexualities from Ganymede to Batman.*

This lack of interest notwithstanding, the Jungian community is a rather receptive place for the analysis and training of gay and lesbian people. Despite the sexist and patriarchal attitudes of its founder, post-Jungian psychology does not regard human sexuality in a normative way and is relatively free from constraints, classification and set patterns (Hauke, 2000; Lingiardi, 2001). What seems to differentiate Jungian institutes from Freudian ones, at least as far as Italy is concerned, is a greater openness to clinical and theoretical changes and less adherence to a psychosexual developmental model. The result is less of a tendency to be directive with patients in treatment. And so, in spite of the fact that one might express more than a suspicion of Jung's homophobia (Hopcke, 1989; Walker, 1991), gay people are not excluded from Jungian societies. The national CIPA conference in 1996, entitled "Femininities/Masculinities: Nostalgia and Reconstruction," was an important moment of discussion on the themes of gender and sexuality for the Italian Jungian community.

LITERATURE REVIEW: THE 1930s TO THE 1970s

In reviewing the general index of the *Rivista di Psicoanalisi*, the journal of the Italian Psychoanalytical Society, there are few articles dealing with homosexuality; those few that have dealt with the subject do so from a narrow perspective. There is a constant linkage of the "homosexual" with psychopathic descriptions or, in the best of cases, with examples of arrested development. In the 30s and 40s, there were no specific contributions about homosexuality. One exception is an article by Emilio Servadio (1932) that re-elaborates the Freudian theory of bisexuality as regards the homosexual component in heterosexuals (Freud, 1905), and the publishing of a psychoanalytic handbook by Cesare Musatti (1949). Musatti's intention was to introduce Freudian psychoanalytic theory, which was then barely known, to the Italian public.[5] In his discussion of homosexuality, Musatti describes Freudian theories without adding any theoretical or clinical contributions of his own.[6]

Among the few references to be found in the 1950s, in 1953, the cultural journal *Ulisse*, in the wake of the American Kinsey Reports on sexual behaviour (Kinsey, Pomeroy and Martin, 1948; Kinsey et al. 1953), published a monographic issue on homosexuality. It attempted to address the subject from every possible point of view: statistical, historical, medical, legal, pedagogical, psychological, and psychoanalytical. Nevertheless, homosexuality is always read in the light of the psychosexual Freudian model. The psychoanalyst Emilio Servadio (1953) focuses on the oral and preoedipal structure and considers homosexuality to be primarily a defense against the psychotic anguish related to early infantile experiences. The neuropsychiatrist Tullio Bazzi (1953) considers homosexuality to be a developmental disorder and expressed skepticism regarding the possibility of modifying it to heterosexuality. On the other hand, Gianfranco Tedeschi (1953), a psychiatrist, considers homosexuality a perversion that can be resolved with psychotherapy.

In the 1960s, the Italian psychoanalytic literature on homosexuality was sparse; it included the contributions of Rubinstein and Lopez (1964) and Bellanova (1965) in the *Rivista di Psicoanalisi*. These contributions are influenced by Kleinian theory, in which the presumed origin of homosexuality shifts to the preoedipal phase and these authors focus on the concept of homosexuality as a defence against psychotic anguish. In May of 1963, a conference in Rome addressed the pathogenic aspects of homosexuality. Noted Italian speakers addressed the biological-constitutional aspects (Gedda, Muscardini), endocrinology (Teodori, Morabito), psychological diagnosis (Ferracuti), and psychopathological and psychiatric issues (Callieri, Frighi). The latter admitted the existence of a small percentage of "normal homosexual" individuals. For the Freudian psychoanalyst Perrotti, homosexuality is the expression of a narcissistic object relationship that renders it similar to a psychotic structure.

In 1968, the "Braibanti Case" drew together many Italian intellectuals in response to government attempts to persecute a homosexual. The leftist intellectual, Aldo Braibanti, was condemned to nine years imprisonment for plagiarism, which was a serious crime at the time and only removed from the Italian penal code a few years later. The severity of the penalty may have been related to the fact that Braibanti was also accused of morally subjugating a 24-year-old man with whom he was having a romantic relationship; the latter was eventually hospitalized in a psychiatric facility where he underwent ECT and received insulin shock therapy. There was a mobilization against Braibanti's conviction on the part of intellectuals and civil libertarians, amongst whom were included the film director Pier Paolo Pasolini and the psychoanalyst Cesare Musatti. This was the first time in Italian history that there was such a public mobilization of intellectuals which dealt directly with homosexual issues.

In the 1970s, as a result of political and cultural battles, a significant change had occurred in Italian society. The gay rights organizations, Collettivi Omosessuali [Homosexual Collectives] and Fronte Unitario Omosessuali Rivoluzionari Italiani [The United Front of Italian Revolutionary Homosexuals] (FUORI)[7] appeared on the scene. Their very appearance brings the psychiatric and psychoanalytic debate into the public arena. In April 1971, the Torinese newspaper, *La Stampa*, published an article entitled "The Unhappy One Who Adores His Own Image: A Problem of Burning Relevance" by Professor Romero, a neurologist at the Mauriziano Hospital in Turin. In a compendium of antihomosexual prejudices which he presents as scientific data, he concludes that "The homosexual, if backed by a desire to be cured, can be, efficiently, by undergoing psychoanalytic therapy." In that same period, the Italian newsweekly, *Panorama*, published a survey of homosexuals who came out of the closet, which included the famous philosopher, Gianni Vattimo. In 1972, at an *International Congress on Deviancy* organized by the Italian Catholic Sexology Centre, various therapies for "curing" homosexuality are proposed, from hypnosis to medial ventricular nucleotomy.

On the psychoanalytic front during the 1970s, there is no movement away from pathological conceptions. On the contrary, the psychoanalyst Franco Fornari (then President of the Italian Psychoanalytic Society and Director of the Psychoanalytic Institute of Literature and Philosophy at Milan University) published *Genitality and Culture* (1975a), a critical review of the Freudian sexual theory. Fornari writes as a confirmed believer in the transformative possibilities of psychoanalysis and of its ethical and political functions. He also takes his beliefs to a wider public as his articles "Homosexuality and Culture" (1975b) and "The Difficult Different Love" (1975c) appear in the Milanese newspaper, *Corriere della Sera*.

Fornari believes that sexuality is a force of nature that must be symbolized, and that this symbolization can take place in ways that are more or less adequate. From his perspective, sexual disorders are seen as "defective symbol-ization"–a kind of neurotic symptom. Fornari maintains that an individual's conflict may be located not only between sexuality and culture (a Freudian concept) but between genitality and pre-genitality as well. He conceptualizes homosexuality as a perversion resulting from confusion over and denial of the dependence on the genital object and an idealization of the pre-genital object. He writes:

> Disregarding anal intercourses that may intervene in homosexual rela-tionships, the inversion seems to be produced over and above the bodily confusion, the confusion of persons, both in relation to the self or the non-self . . . The homosexual builds up a fundamentally narcissistic rela-tionship, a denial of his own separateness both from his mother and his partner . . . It is about a pre-genital culture, founded on symbolic equa-tion, instead of the true symbolization. (Fornari, 1975a, pp. 27-28, our translation)

In 1977, Mario Mieli publishes "Elements of Homosexual Criticism."[8] Mieli, *enfant-prodige en travesti* and biting intellectual, was a unique figure in the Italian cultural world of the 1970s: well-bred, *bourgoise*, militant, radical communist and dandy, he committed suicide at the age of thirty. Mieli fero-ciously and "brazenly" fought against antihomosexual biases. Accepting the Freudian theory of polymorphous perversity and universal bisexuality as a starting point, Mieli accuses society of being repressive towards children, of performing a kind of "educative castration." The aim is to force children to re-move those sexual tendencies judged by society to be perverse. In other words, the objective of edu-castration is to transform the polymorphous perverse child into a heterosexual adult, whose eroticism is mutilated but conforms with the norm. The repression of homosexuality determines the rejection of the open expressions of gay desire on the part of society. Mieli takes issue with the for-mulations like those below of Fornari from *Homosexuality and Culture:*

> The homosexual identifies himself with his own mother and imagines his own partner as a substitute of himself as a child. . . . The homosexual not only wants to retrieve in an autarchic way a relationship of childish love that is irretrievable, but does it by way of semantic confusion, like Narcissus, who mistakes his own reflection in the stream for another. (Fornari, 1975a, our translation)

Mieli accuses Fornari of speaking haphazardly, insofar as homosexuals are the only ones who know what it is to be a homosexual.[9] Mieli insists on the universal presence of the homoerotic desire, normally negated by the dominant heterosexual ideology. He claims that as long as homosexuality is repressed, the "homosexual problem" will affect everyone, insofar as gay desire is present in every human being. The homosexuals' liberation is part of human emancipation, inasmuch as the former guarantees the achievement of free communication between human beings, independently of their sex. Although he does not use the term, and it is uncertain if he read Weinberg (1972), Mieli lays out the concept of "internalized homophobia," stating:

> Homosexuals are so induced to think of themselves as sick, that it sometimes happens that they begin to see themselves in this way: our real sickness is that the illusion of illness can make us truly sick. In an analogous way, he/she who has been locked up in a lunatic asylum, may carry the stereotyped signs of facial "folly," that is, traces of persecution and imprisonment, the interiorized "therapy" comes under the form of an illness. (Mieli, 1977, p. 230)

LITERATURE REVIEW:
THE 1980s TO THE PRESENT

In the 1980s, three articles on homosexuality appeared in the *Rivista Sperimentale di Freniatria*. The first, by two psychologists, Angelini and Macciò (1980), reports the results of a research experiment aimed at determining, through the use of figure drawing tests, what differences, if any, exist between male and female homosexuality. The second paper by two psychiatrists, Bizzarri and Onano (1982), viewed homosexuality as a defense from psychotic disintegration. The final paper by a psychoanalyst, Nobili (1983), contains similar arguments to a 1983 article by Zucconi, that appeared in the psychoanalytic journal *Gli Argonauti*. According to both authors, the prejudice coming from so-called normality traps homosexuals into the impossibility of ever being free from . . . their illness! Passi Tognazzo and Baratella (1981) try to find out, with the Rorschach test, well-grounded indications for diagnosing homosexuality. In contrast to Hooker's (1957) nonpathological findings, they conclude that the test brings out a lack of sexual identification and a conflictual relationship with the father. The hypnotist and psychologist Fabiano (1981) writes of "A Case of Female Homosexuality Resolved in Five Hypnotherapy Sessions" which appears to say it all! Angelini et al. (1983) propose some criteria for the cure of homosexuality: motivation for change, age of 35 or under, and previous satisfactory heterosexual relationships.

In the beginning of the eighties, the Centro Milanese di Psicoanalisi organized a panel on sexual disorders. Speaking from an alternative perspective, in her 1983 report, Argentieri (personal communication) speaks of the complexity of the homosexual problem, which cannot be considered as a psychological state or syndrome. In the "Textbook of Psychoanalysis" (Semi, 1989), a chapter dedicated to perversions reads:

> A special status should be granted to homosexuality, nearer to neurosis, because of its relatively mature structure, so much so that on the part of many authors there is now a tendency to exclude it from the field of perversions, in the strict sense of the word. (De Martis, 1989, p. 262)

De Martis, who adheres to Freudian psychosexual theory, recognizes different kinds of homosexuality: latent; Oedipal; "social" (as a basis for satisfactory friendships and social contact, i.e., army, church, etc.); conflicting and prevalently ego-dystonic (with self-blame and impulsive behaviours); re-actualizing an insufficiently genitalized sexuality (occurring in immature personalities); and finally, he lists "the homosexual behaviour of the gay activists." The author wonders whether this last behavior should be considered perverted, or whether it should be seen as an expression of one of the infinite variants of human nature. The author nevertheless tends to underline the pathological aspect; for De Martis, homosexuality is often the tip of the iceberg of a much more complex perverse structure. The paper ends with a reference to homosexuality as an expression of a psychotic condition, as in the case of Schreber (Freud, 1911), serving a dual role: unbridled and protective. The "psychotic aspect" of homosexuality is reasserted by Arrigoni Scortecci (1989), following Bak (1946) (paranoia and homosexuality) and the Kleinian authors (homosexuality as a defense against persecutory figures).

While the psychoanalytic mainstream pathologized homosexuality, the journal *Rivista di Psicoterapia e Scienze Umane*, directed by Pier Francesco Galli, took a different editorial position and presented normative, psychoanalytic views of homosexuality. Amongst the authors published are Morgenthaler (1982), Moor (1985, 1989) and, more recently, Drescher (1996). Then, towards the end of the 80s and the beginning of the 90s, thanks in part to the diffusion in Italy of the contributions of American relational psychoanalysts (Mitchell, 1978, 1981), the journal *Psychoanalytic Dialogues*, and of gay and gender studies (for example, the journals *Gender & Psychoanalysis* and *Studies in Gender and Sexuality*), the attitude of Italian psychoanalysts began to change. For the first time, some Italian psychoanalysts proposed a new vision of homosexuality, starting to amend a series of theoretical and morally prejudicial errors.[10] A public occasion occurs in 1996 with the Italian translation of the American Richard Isay's first book, *Being Homosexual*. He is presented to an Italian audience by the psychoanalysts Barale, De Masi, Savoia and Lingiardi, and the book was reviewed by De Masi (1996) in the *Rivista di Psicoanalisi*. The Freudian community realizes that "gay psychoanalysts" exist and can write openly!

In the early 1990s, the *Rivista di Sessuologia* made a tentative start and published some innovative articles on both the theoretical and clinical level, but particularly on the sociocultural one (Bigagli, 1992a, 1992b; Casonato, 1993; D'Ascenzio, Venturelli and Manfrina, 1993; Ghizzani, 1993). The psychologist and University Professor Anna Oliverio Ferraris (1994) declared the necessity of referring to homosexualities and bisexualities in the plural, and not in a pathologizing way.

For the Freudians in the 1990s, however, it was still a hard climb. In 1992, in the *Rivista di Psicoanalisi*, Petrella published "Explorations in the Cities of the Plain: The Homosexual in Analysis." There, six cases are discussed, all of which are individuals who had not entered analysis to cure their homosexuality. Although Petrella specifies that his observations are related to his narrow clinical experience, he nevertheless transmits a generalized pathological view of homosexuality per se. According to Petrella, the compulsive sexual conduct of his patients is indispensable to avoid the development of anxiety, and in this sense bears characteristics similar to those of drug dependency. He observes that even if the homosexual patient does not ask to be "cured," nevertheless at a certain stage in treatment he wants the analyst to declare where he stands upon this issue. In Petrella's opinion, homosexuality should not be "respected," but should always be analyzed. He adds: "Patients are afraid of normalization as they depreciate normalcy, because they have narcissistically cathected their position, the relinquishing of which would expose them to the experiences of terrifying emptiness and loss and to a confrontation with a radical conflict from which they have fled through homosexuality" (1992, p. 912). In other words, Petrella considers homosexuality to be the result of a defensive unconscious organization, with its conscious component as potentially ego-syntonic. The functions of the homosexual object seem to consist in bringing about–instantaneously and on command–the reinforcement of an identity which is threatened and on the brink of collapse. For Petrella, homosexuality cannot be considered either a nosographic term nor a stable outcome of conflicting constellations. It is, instead, a symptom related to primal phantasies, which have to be analyzed in metapsychological terms.[11] Petrella's views show that even in the 1990s, even the most brilliant of psychoanalysts had difficulty regarding homosexuality as an expression of affectivity and human sexuality. This tradition continues in the journal *Gli Argonauti* where Bennati and Zucconi (1997) and then again Bennati (1999) continue to stress a pathological concept of homosexuality.

In "Reflections on the Undecidable," Badoni (1998) asks herself why some psychoanalysts, when they have a homosexual patient in analysis, tend to clinically define him/her according to his/her orientation.[12] Badoni focuses on the countertransference of the analyst: the conflation of sexual orientation with pathology when the homosexuality is ego-dystonic, and from an opposite direction, the collusion between analyst and patient not to analyze the sexual orientation. But in treating a sexual orientation, whether homo or hetero, as interwoven in the organization of the personality, one risks not integrating the sexuality with the personality. To get over what she sees as a paradox, Badoni suggests the "undecidable," the necessity of floating suspended over this matter until the patient finds his or her own way to strenghten his or her identity. However Badoni's work does not seem to take in consideration the existence of patients who turn to analysis with a well-defined homosexual identity. In "Homosexuality: A Term Too Vague and at the Same Time Too Reductive," Savoia (1998) is perhaps the first Italian Freudian analyst to discuss homosexuality without defensive or psychopathological meanings, but simply as a congenital form of sexuality. She affirms that a specific, homosexual, psychological typology does not exist. She also underscores the role of social homophobia and denounces the lack of a model of normal homosexual development in psychoanalysis.

The 1990s saw the publication of various volumes on homosexuality. In addition to Lingiardi's (1997) aforementioned book, and his postscript to Isay's (1996) book, there are: *Different Identities: The Psychology of Homosexuality* (Del Favero and Palomba, 1996); *The Worst Offence* (Pietrantoni, 1999); *Psychotherapy with Homosexual Clients* (Montano, 2000). Cognitively and social psychologically oriented, the latter three books primarily focus on homophobia, educational approaches and psychotherapy. The psychiatrist Rigliano (2001) has recently published *Love Without Scandal* in which he underscores the way homosexuality should be read–not so much from the perspective of sexual behavior, but from the quality of an individual's affective relationships.

In the Italian psychoanalytic literature it is still necessary to turn to translations of foreign contributors, since Italian psychoanalysts, except for the ones quoted above, continue to avoid exposing themselves on this theme. Bassi and Galli (2000) have recently edited an anthology, *Homosexuality and Psychoanalysis*, that brings together contributions from Parin, Moss, Moor, Drescher, Isay, Blechner, Phillips, and two early, historical papers by Fritz Morgenthaler and Stephen A. Mitchell.

Nevertheless, attitudes are beginning to change in both the Italian Psychoanalytic Society and in the National Training Institute. There are now various groups within those organizations who are reflecting upon, on both a clinical and theoretical level, the contradictions and limits of psychoanalysis on the subject of homosexuality. For example, in the Milanese Center for Psychoanalysis, Capozzi and De Masi have started a study group on homosexuality. Their belief is that the absence of a psychoanalytical theory contemplating the existence of a "normal" homosexuality illustrates the limits of the literature reviewed up to this point.[13]

PSYCHIATRY AND PSYCHOLOGY TEXTBOOKS: A BRIEF REVIEW

Up until the seventies, most psychiatric textbooks listed homosexuality among psychopathic sexual states (Morselli, 1915; Moglie, 1930; Gozzano, 1958); others considered it in a more generic way as a "sexual disorder with perverse characteristics," as in the *Textbook of Psychiatry* by Bini and Bazzi (1967). The latter, in its 1971 revised version, defines homosexuality as an incomplete sexual development due to a fragile ego. Scoppa's *Psychiatric Medicine* (1978) also links homosexuality to psychopathy.

In the eighties and early nineties, textbooks primarily described homosexuality as a condition of low statistical frequency, with a consequent diagnostic tendency towards the concept of deviance (Giberti and Rossi, 1986; Reda, 1993). During the same period, Sarteschi and Maggini (1989) linked homosexuality to personality disorders.

Other textbooks in this period, however, began to take alternative positions; for example, Balestrieri (1986) underlines how so-called psychopathology is, in many cases, linked to feelings of guilt and shame. In the *Dictionary of Psychology*, Galimberti (1992) describes various theoretical viewpoints, including one that considers homosexuality to be "normal." In the *Italian Textbook of Psychiatry*, Pancheri and Cassano (1992, 1999), following the DSM classification system, describe "a form of" ego-syntonic homosexuality as a normal variant of sexual behaviour, but nevertheless they still describe homosexuality as always being a pathological condition. A similar, double edged formulation is offered in the *Handbook of Psychiatry* by Fossi and Pallanti (1994) who admit that "homosexuals" show no greater evidence of psychiatric disorders than heterosexuals–even though homosexuality is a pathological condition!

Even at the end of the nineties, Italian psychiatric attitudes toward "homosexuality" remained controversial. In *Dynamic Psychiatry and Psychopathology*, Montanari (1996) defines the "homosexual" as a person affected by an identity problem. Invernizzi (1996) follows the DSM-IV classification closely and, therefore, in his manual the term homosexuality simply does not appear. The same is true for Vella (1994), Penati (1994) and Gaston and Gaston (1997). Nevertheless, Lalli's (1999) handbook anachronistically considers homosexuality to be a sexual deviation.

HOMOSEXUALITY AND PSYCHOANALYSIS IN ITALY: PRELIMINARY NOTES FROM AN ONGOING RESEARCH PROJECT

In the course of the writing of this article, the authors initiated an empirical research project with the aim of obtaining a picture of contemporary Italian psychoanalytic attitudes towards homosexuality. The most representative Italian psychoanalytic institutes (SPI, AIPsi, CIPA, AIPA and ISIPSé)[14] were selected and members of each institutes were sent a questionnaire.[15] Here, are reported some preliminary findings:[16]

a. Of 600 questionnaires sent out, 206 replies were received;[17]
b. There was no significant correlation between the gender of the analyst and the analyst's attitudes towards homosexuality. A less pathologizing attitude that, at first glance, seems to characterize the female sample is linked to a higher rate of "I don't know" answers;
c. There was a significant correlation between a more pathologizing attitude of homosexual and respondents having a medical degree. In addition, the SPI-AIPsi members (that is the members of the Freudian societies) are more pathologizing than the AIPA-CIPA members (that is the members of the Jungian societies);
d. In comparison to the Jungian sample, the Freudian respondents were more likely to adhere to evolutionary theories which regard homosexuality as a pathological condition. Moreover, the majority of the Freudian sample does not believe that an "out homosexual" can be a psychoanalyst, let alone a training analyst;
e. Finally, Freudian psychoanalysts recognize in their institutes the existence of a discriminatory policy aimed at discouraging gay and lesbian candidates. It is also interesting to note that a respondent's position in the institute influences the answer: while candidates and members said there was a discriminatory policy, training analysts denied it.[18]

CONCLUSIONS

It can be said, in a general way, that with a lag of about ten years, Italy has followed, even with its local cultural declinations, the attitudes of American mental health professions toward homosexuality. In 1973, the American Psychiatric Association began to consider homosexuality as a normal variation of human sexuality. This position was not officially accepted by the American Psychoanalytic Association until 1991 (Roughton, 1995). In Italy, since the end of World War II to the present, homosexuality has never been psychiatrically labeled in a persecutory way. This comparatively *laissez-faire* approach may explain why Italian medical, psychological and psychoanalytic associations have yet to produce an explicit policy of non-discrimination in their by-laws. For example, it is presently inconceivable that a group such as the Committee on Gay, Lesbian and Bisexual Issues of the American Psychiatric Association could exist in the Italian Psychiatric Association. Everybody would say: "Why do we need a gay and lesbian branch? Gay and lesbian can be whatever they are wherever they want."

The lack of enthusiasm among Italian psychoanalytic societies (and among some other European ones as well) for inserting the non-discrimination statement approved by the APA in 1991, is the clearest example of the "don't ask-don't tell" climate previously described (also see Drescher, 1995, 1998). In fact, many European psychoanalysts consider this attitude the most consistent with an analytical stance. They maintain that the task of the analytic treatment is to evaluate the candidate in her/his wholeness, to understand her/his affectivity and sexuality and the capacity for healthy and satisfaying relationships. However, this position seems either hypocritical or, even worse, a disavowal of the existence of antihomosexual bias. As the aforementioned research project seems to indicate, everyone knows there are no openly gay or lesbian psychoanalysts in the International Psychoanalytic Association (IPA) affiliated Italian societies. As Roughton (2001) notes, if there is no antihomosexual prejudice, then why are there no gay or lesbian psychoanalysts?

Mitchell (1996) has noted that in the analytic literature, a typical response to the problems raised by the patients' sexual orientation has always been the notion of psychoanalytic "neutrality":

> . . . stay out of it and let the patient find his or her own way. But that guide is not as helpful as it once was. There has been a broad movement in virtually all contemporary analytic schools of thought in the direction of understanding psychoanalysis in interactive terms, in which the analyst is now regarded as having a considerable impact on the process, both conscious and unconscious, both intended and unintended. Given the current array of possibilities, even the analyst's choice of theories with regard to gender and sexual orientation must be seen to reflect the analyst's own dynamics and personality in some fashion. In working with gender and sexuality, the analyst's own preferences and values must be taken into account, reflected upon, and weighted. (pp. 48-49)

The lack of an Italian psychoanalytic literature which regards homosexuality as non-pathological strengthens the impression that there exist antihomosexual biases. Moreover, in the Italian psychoanalytic literature, even between 1950 and 1980, there is also a total lack of clinical studies of patients "directed" to change their sexual orientation. There is also a lack of literature on any satisfying analyses of gay and lesbian individuals. In contrast to the American experience, there is no Italian tradition of autobiographical reports of psychoanalytic or psychiatric experiences of attempts to cure one's homosexuality (Duberman, 1991; Isay, 1996). All this seems consistent with the "don't ask, don't tell" attitude previously described.

There are, however, anecdotes and personal communications of patients who have undergone what Mitchell (1981) calls directive-suggestive therapies, and accounts of young doctors or psychologists who were dissuaded from taking up psychiatric or psychoanalytic trainings. There are also anecdotes of patients requesting psychoanalytic therapy to change their sexual orientation and of psychoanalysts who have accepted that request at face value without exploring its many possible meanings. For example, a well-known Milanese psychoanalyst looked perplexed at a young gay man who had asked him to begin an analysis and said, "You know, homosexuality is a lid–it always hides something." Another young patient, troubled by homosexual dreams, was told, "The problem is that you are afraid of women." An adolescent patient tells his therapist that he's fallen in love with a male school friend, and she, with a reassuring smile replies, "Don't worry, it happens to everyone during adolescence. You'll see, soon you'll be in love with a beautiful girl!" A lesbian at the end of her first consultation was told by the analyst, "I am sorry, I cannot take you in analysis as I don't know anything about homosexuality." The woman felt the analyst regarded homosexuality as an exotic disease.

Similar attitudes exist when analysts speak to each other. At a panel on "Psychoanalysis and Homosexuality" attended by one of the authors, one panelist remarked, "We all have a homosexual component–but we must succeed in sublimating it!" A gay psychiatrist, at the end of a personal analysis, was to undergo admission interviews for training at a psychoanalytic institute. His analyst cautioned him not to mention a word about his homosexuality. The candidate told his analyst that to do so would be placing all of his analytic work to date in a questionable light. The analyst reassured him, saying "it is a stupid thing to risk a career for a formality." The psychiatrist appeared before the examiners. During the interview, the questions became more and more personal. The candidate started to talk about an imaginary girl he is dating. Eventually, the interview fell apart and he was not admitted to the institute. Certainly the candidate was very confused about himself. But what about the analyst? (Lingiardi, 2001).

It has taken psychoanalysts many years to understand that words and attitudes like these can cause severe damage to the psychic equilibrium of their patients. However, some psychoanalysts still do not seem to recognize the importance of the role they could play in helping their gay and lesbian patients achieve a positive sense of self through acceptance of their sexual orientation. For a long period of time, gay people didn't trust psychoanalysis because of their fear of being obliged to question the normality of their sexual orientation and consequently the integrity of their personal identity. Now that the cultural climate and clinical attitudes are changing, gay and lesbian people have begun to reapproach the analytic consulting room. However, apart from the more gay and lesbian-friendly Jungian Associations, Freudian institutes don't seem quite ready to accept homosexual members. Drescher's (1996; in Bassi and Galli, 2000, p. 88) words fit the Italian situation when he writes that for many heterosexuals "the absence of openly gay voices is part of everyday psychoanalytic life. But to the small gay analytic community, the silence appears deafening." "Silence," continues Drescher, "is a symbol of indifference, and indifference a special kind of disdain. Let us say that the exclusive theorizing of heterosexuals about homosexuality is as meaningful as had been the male theorizing on female sexuality." Elsewhere, Drescher (1995, p. 240) notes, "The history of antihomosexual bias illustrates the point that it is extremely difficult to separate a scientific theory from the cultural matrix in which theories are formulated." Highlighting this Italian history permits us to see how discrimination operates: "usually behind closed doors, often insidiously, and ultimately corrupting the ideals of the institutions in which it flourishes."

NOTES

1. When Italy was on its way to becoming a unified nation, in 1861, the criminal code of Northern Italy was extended to the rest of the country. However, the law that punished homosexual acts was not extended to Southern Italy, giving birth to a "double standard." In 1889, the Zanardelli Code was promulgated–the first of unified Italy–which finally decriminalized homosexual relationships between consenting adults, at least privately and without public scandal: "It was enough not to make too much noise and to consume in silence this venial mortal sin" (Rossi Barilli, 1999, p. 4).

2. Musatti was forbidden to teach after Italy's Fascist regime's racial laws were enacted.

3. In the summer of 1931, the analysis was interrupted because of Weiss's move from Trieste to Rome.

4. The passage at issue may be the one in which Freud said "in general, undertaking to transform a fully developed homosexual into a heterosexual does not offer any more a chance of success than to undertake the opposite; the only difference is that this latter, for very good reasons of a practical nature, is never attempted" (Freud, 1920, p. 151).

5. In Italy, the translation of the complete works of Freud only took place in the 1970s.

6. In spite of his liberal political opinions, Musatti was not open to any of the new ideas that were developing in international psychoanalysis.

7. "FUORI" in Italian means "OUT."

8. For an American interpretation of Mieli, see Dean and Lane (2001).

9. When challenged by a group of gay activists at his own university, Fornari declares, "Homosexuals cannot impede me from carrying out my university duties by demanding a debate on a subject that has nothing to do with my course: it's as if a group of delicatessen owners interrupted my lesson to discuss ham and salami." Mieli (1977, p. 200) "interprets" the association used by Fornari between ham and salami and homosexuals in a highly ironic manner: "If ham and salami are pork meats, thereby 'piggish,' the association for Fornari is that homosexuals cannot be allowed to interrupt a lecture on psychology and demand a debate–because of their 'piggish' nature."

10. In those years, the Institute of Politics, Economics and Social Studies (ISPES, 1991) in collaboration with the gay association Arci-Gay, published the most complete research ever conducted on the homosexual condition in Italy. This research aims at analyzing two aspects: (a) the experience of 300 homosexual persons and (b) Italians' perception of homosexuality. Recently, the sociologists Barbagli and Colombo (2001) published a new survey (more than 3,000 of people interviewed, the largest research project of this kind in Europe) on the gay and lesbian condition in Italy.

11. In his cases, Petrella writes of the centrality of a catastrophic childhood anguish, that in being held back has determined a strong limitation of the ego and formation of symptoms. The defensive, compulsive behaviour that Petrella describes is, in fact, found in borderline or psychotic patients, in whom the compulsive search for the (homo-or-hetero) sexual object serves to avoid panic and anguish, but does not seem to be specific to the homosexual person.

12. Magee and Miller (1997) identify this tendency within psychoanalysis as synecdoche, a grammatical term in which the part stands for the whole.

13. Homosexualities, male and female, imply different structures and lead to complex clinical situations with a variety of possibilities that, similar to the situation with heterosexual patients, must be recognized and gone into in depth. Psychoanalytic theory is not yet equipped to understand fully how imagination and sexual choice develop and which factors are brought into play.

14. SPI (Società Italiana di Psicoanalisi [Italian Psychoanalytic Society]); AIPsi (Associazione Italiana di Psicoanalisi [Italian Psychoanalytic Association]); CIPA (Centro Italiano di Psicologia Analitica [Italian Society for Analytical Psychology]); AIPA (Associazione Italiana di Psicologia Analitica [Italian Association for Analytical Psychology]); ISIPSé (Istituto di Specializzazione in Psicologia Psicoanalitica del Sé e Psuicoanalisi Relazionale [Institute for the Specialization in Psychoanalytic Self-Psychology and Relational Psychoanalysis]).

15. The questionnaire requested the filling in of an initial informative selection relative to personal data: sex, age, place of origin, degree, membership of societies, qualification within the society, theory, models for reference. The second section is composed of 13 items (amongst them: "I believe that psychoanalysis has a valid theory to explain the genesis of male and female homosexuality"; "I believe that a good psychoanalytical therapy must help the homosexual patient become heterosexual"; "I think that homosexuality is an expression of pathological family dynamics and I tend to consider homosexuality as a symptom"; "I think that an openly homosexual psychoanalyst can be a valid colleague"; "I think that in the psychoanalytic society/association I belong to there exists a discriminatory policy aimed at discouraging candidates who declare openly that they are homosexual or bisexual").

16. The results of this research project, conducted by the authors together with Maria Grazia Acquaviva and Monica Luci, will be the subject of a future publication.

17. This response rate in itself may indicate the avoidant/dismissive attitude around the subject.

18. A study conducted by members of the American Psychoanalytical Association (MacIntosh, 1994) found that 97.6% (90.5% in our sample) of them did not believe that "the homosexual patients can or should change their sexual orientation into a heterosexual one." Yet, 34.4% thought that "most of the other analysts believe that homosex-

ual patients can or should change their sexual orientation to a heterosexual one." We read this statistic as sign of a divergence between what psychoanalysts think and what they do.

REFERENCES

Aldrich, R. (1993), *The Seduction of the Mediterranean*. New York: Routledge.

Angelini, C. & Macciò, A.M. (1980), *Il Sé psicosessuale nell'omosessualità* [The psychosexual self in homosexuality]. *Rivista Sperimentale di Freniatria*, 104(2): 237-276.

Angelini, G., Viotti, M., Governa, R., Olivero, C. & Sabbatini, F. (1983), *Omosessualità oggi* [Homosexuality today]. *Rivista Internazionale di Psicologia e Ipnosi*, 24(1): 85-91.

Arrigoni Scortecci, M. (1989), *La costruzione di modelli psicoanalitici nelle psicosi* [The construction of psychoanalytical models in the psychoses]. In: *Trattato di Psicoanalisi* [*Textbook of Psychoanalysis*], ed. A. A. Semi. Milano: Raffaello Cortina, pp. 621-690.

Badoni, M. (1998), *Riflessioni sull'indecidibile* [Reflections on the undecidable]. *Rivista di Psicoanalisi*, XLIV(2):213-233.

Bak, R.C. (1946), Masochism in paranoia. *Psychoanal. Quart.*, 15:285-301.

Balestrieri, A. (1986), *Trattato di psichiatria* [*Textbook of Psychiatry*]. Roma: Il Pensiero Scientifico.

Barbagli, M. & Colombo, A. (2001), *Omosessuali moderni. Gay e lesbiche in Italia* [*Contemporary Homosexuals: Gays and Lesbians in Italy*]. Bologna: Il Mulino.

Bassi, F. & Galli, P.F., eds. (2000), *L'omosessualità nella psicoanalisi* [*Homosexuality and Psychoanalysis*]. Torino: Einaudi.

Bazzi, T. (1953), *L'omosessualità e la psicoterapia* [Homosexuality and psychotherapy]. *Ulisse*, 3(18):646-656.

Bellanova, P. (1965), *Rapporti tra terapia ed espressione pittorica nell'analisi di un omosessuale* [The relationship between therapy and expressive painting in the analysis of a homosexual]. *Rivista Italiana di Psicoanalisi*, XI(3): 211-225.

Bennati, P. (1999), *Femminile e maschile: l'incontro?* [Female and male: The encounter?]. *Gli Argonauti*, 83:315-319.

Bennati, P. & Zucconi, S. (1997), *Un gioco da ragazzi* [A boys' game]. *Gli Argonauti*, 72:95-103.

Bigagli, A. (1992a), *Per una identità etero- omo-e bisessuale* [Towards a hetero-, homo- and bisexual identity]. *Rivista di Sessuologia*, 16(2):28-33.

Bigagli, A. (1992b), *L'immagine dell'omosessualità nella stampa italiana* [The image of homosexuality in the Italian press]. *Rivista di Sessuologia*, 16(2):169-185.

Bini, L. & Bazzi, T. (1971), *Trattato di psichiatria* [Textbook of psychiatry]. Milano: Vallardi.

Bizzarri, C. & Onano, R. (1982), *Omosessualità come difesa dalla disgregazione psicotica* [Homosexuality as a defense against psychotic disgregation]. *Rivista Sperimentale di Freniatria*, 106(6):1289-1312.

Carotenuto, A. (1982), *Il diverso* [The different one]. *Giornale Storico di Psicologia Dinamica*, 6(12):3-19.

Carotenuto, A. (1985), *L'autunno della coscienza* [*The Autumn of Counsciousness*]. Torino: Boringhieri.

Casonato M. (1993), *La sessualità maschile, femminile, omosessuale: teorie e modelli psicoanalitici* [Male, female and homosexual sexuality: Psychoanalytic theories and models]. *Rivista di sessuologia*, 17(1):7-20.

D'Ascenzio, I., Venturelli, M. & Manfrina, G. (1993), *Diagnosi e Terapia nell'omosessualità femminile. Una prospettiva relazionale* [Diagnosis and treatment of female homosexuality: A relational perspective]. *Rivista di Sessuologia*, 17(1):21-24.

De Martis, D. (1989), *La perversione. Aspetti generali* [Perversion: General aspects]. In: *Trattato di psicoanalisi* [*Textbook of Psychoanalysis*], ed. A. A. Semi. Milano: Raffaello Cortina, pp. 255-284.

De Masi, F. (1996), *Recensione a "Essere Omosessuali," di R. Isay* [Review of "Being Homosexual," by R. Isay]. *Rivista di Psicoanalisi*, XLII(3):491-495.

Dean, T. & Lane C., eds. (2001), *Homosexuality and Psychoanalysis*. Chicago, IL: University of Chicago Press.

Del Favero, R. & Palomba, M. (1996), *Identità diverse: la psicologia dell'omosessualità* [*Different Identities: The Psychology of Homosexuality*]. Roma: Kappa Edizioni.

Downing, C. (1991), *Myths and Mysteries of Same-Sex Love*. New York: Continuum Press.

Drescher, J. (1995), Anti-homosexual bias in training. In: *Disorienting Sexualities*, ed. T. Domenici & R. C. Lesser. New York: Routledge, pp. 227-241.

Drescher, J. (1996), *Atteggiamenti psicoanalitici verso l'omosessualità* [Psychoanalytic attitudes toward homosexuality]. *Psicoterapia e Scienze Umane*, 30(2):5-24. Reprinted in: *L'omosessualità nella psicoanalisi* [*Homosexuality in Psychoanalysis*], ed. F. Bassi & P. F. Galli. Torino: Einaudi, 2000, pp. 67-88.

Drescher, J. (1998), *Psychoanalytic Therapy and the Gay Man*. Hillsdale, NJ: The Analytic Press.

Duberman, M. (1991), *Cures: A Gay Man's Odyssey*. New York: Dutton.

Fabiano, G. (1981), *Un caso di omosessualità femminile risolto in cinque sedute ipnoterapeutiche* [A case of female homosexuality resolved in five hypnotherapy sessions]. *Rivista Internazionale di Psicologia e Ipnosi*, 22(1):45-48.

Fornari, F. (1975a), *Genitalità e cultura* [Genitality and Culture]. Milano: Feltrinelli.

Fornari, F. (1975b), *Omosessualità e cultura* [Homosexuality and culture]. *Corriere della Sera*, February 12, p. 3.

Fornari, F. (1975c), *Il difficile amore diverso* [The difficult, different love]. *Corriere della Sera*, November 12.

Fossi, G. & Pallanti, S. (1994), *Manuale di psichiatria* [*Handbook of Psychiatry*]. Milano: CEA.

Freud, S. (1905), Three essays on the theory of sexuality. *Standard Edition*, 7:123-246. London: Hogarth Press, 1953.

Freud, S. (1911), Psycho-analytic notes on an autobiographical account of a case of paranoia. *Standard Edition*, 12:1-82. London: Hogarth Press, 1958.

Freud, S. (1920), The psychogenesis of a case of homosexuality in a woman. *Standard Edition*, 18:145-172. London: Hogarth Press, 1955.

Freud, S. (1935), Anonymous (Letter to an American mother). In: *The Letters of Sigmund Freud*, ed. E. Freud, 1960. New York: Basic Books, pp. 423-424.

Galimberti, U. (1992), *Dizionario di psicologia [Dictionary of Psychology]*. Torino: UTET.

Gaston, A. & Gaston, C.M. (1997), *Psichiatria e igiene mentale* [Psychiatry and Mental Health]. Milano: Masson.

Ghizzani, A. (1993), *Quali disagi e quali terapie nei problemi dell'orientamento sessuale?* [Which impairments and which therapies in sexual orientation problems?]. *Rivista di Sessuologia*, 17(1):25-30.

Giberti, F. & Rossi, R. (1986), *Manuale di psichiatria [Handbook of Psychiatry]*. Second Edition. Milano: La Nuova Libraria.

Gozzano, M. (1958), *Compendio di psichiatria [Handbook of Psychiatry]*. Torino: Rosemberg & Sellier.

Hauke, C. (2000), *Jung and the Postmodern*. London: Routledge.

Hillman, J. (1972), *The Myth of Analysis: Three Essays in Archetypal Psychology*. Evanston, IL: Northwestern University Press.

Hillman, J. (1991), *A Blue Fire: Selected Writings of James Hillman*, ed. T. Moore. New York: Harper Perennial.

Hooker, E. (1957), The adjustment of the male overt homosexual. *J. Proj. Tech*, 21:18-31.

Hopcke, R. (1989), *Jung, Jungians & Homosexuality*. Boston, MA: Shambhala.

Invernizzi, G. (1996), *Manuale di psichiatria e psicologia clinica [Handbook of Psychiatry and Clinical Psychology]*. Milano: McGraw-Hill.

Isay, R. (1989), *Being Homosexual: Gay Men and Their Development*. New York: Farrar, Straus and Giroux. Translated as *Essere omosessuali*. Milano: Raffaello Cortina Editore, 1996.

Isay, R. (1996), *Becoming Gay: The Journey to Self-Acceptance*. New York: Pantheon.

ISPES (*Istituto di Studi Politici Economici e Sociali*) (1991), *Il sorriso di Afrodite. Rapporto sulla condizione omosessuale in Italia [Aphrodite's Smile: Report on the Homosexual Condition in Italy]*. Edited by C. Fiore. Firenze: Vallecchi.

Kinsey, A., Pomeroy, W. & Martin, C. (1948), *Sexual Behavior in the Human Male*. Philadelphia, PA: Saunders.

Kinsey, A., Pomeroy, W., Martin, C. & Gebhard, P. (1953), *Sexual Behavior in the Human Female*. Philadelphia, PA: Saunders.

Kirsch, T.B. (2000), *The Jungians: A Comparative Historical Perspective*. London: Routledge.

Lalli, N. (1999), *Manuale di psichiatria e psicoterapia [Handbook of Psychiatry and Psychotherapy]*. Napoli: Liguori.

Lavagetto, A., ed. (1981), *Per conoscere Saba [Knowing Saba]*. Milan: Mondadori.

Lingiardi, V. (1995), *Omosessualità: sintomo, relazione d'oggetto, individuazione* [Homosexuality: Symptom, object relation, individuation]. *La Pratica Analitica*, 12:113-128.

Lingiardi, V. (1996), *L'omosessualità mito psicoanalitico e corredo genetico* [Homosexuality: Psychoanalytic myth and genetic complement]. In: *Essere omosessuali*, by R. Isay. Milano: Raffaello Cortina Editore, pp. 123-137.

Lingiardi, V. (1997), *Compagni D'Amore: Da Ganimede a Batman: Identità e Mito nelle Omossesualità Maschili*. Milano, Italy: Raffaello Cortina. Translated as *Men in Love: Male Homosexualities from Ganymede to Batman*. Chicago: Open Court, 2002.

Lingiardi, V. (2001), Ars erotica or scientia sexualis? Post-Jungian reflections on the homosexualities. *J. Gay & Lesb. Psychother.*, 5(1):29-57.

Lucchini, C. (1997), *L'esperienza analitica a confronto con i percorsi tardo moderni nella soggettività maschile* [Psychoanalytic experience with late modern paths in male subjectivity]. *La Pratica Analitica*, 16:7-14.

MacIntosh, H. (1994), Attitudes and experiences of psychoanalysts in analyzing homosexual patients. *J. Amer. Psychoanal. Assn.*, 42:1183-1207.

Magee, M. & Miller, D. (1997), *Lesbian Lives: Psychoanalytic Narratives Old and New*. Hillsdale, NJ: The Analytic Press.

Marcovecchio, A., ed. (1983), *La spada d'amore. Lettere scelte (1902-1957) di Umberto Saba* [*Sword of Love. Umberto Saba's Letters, (1902-1957)*]. Milan: Mondadori.

Mieli, M. (1977), *Elementi di critica omosessuale*. Torino: Einaudi. Translated by David Fernbach as *Homosexuality and Liberation: Elements of a Gay Critique*. London: Gay Men's, 1980.

Mitchell, S.A. (1978), Psychodynamics, homosexuality, and the question of pathology. *Psychiat.*, 41:254-263.

Mitchell, S.A. (1981), The psychoanalytic treatment of homosexuality: Some technical considerations. *Internat. Rev. Psycho-Anal.*, 8:63-80.

Mitchell, S.A. (1996), Gender and sexual orientation in the age of post-modernism: The plight of the perplexed clinician. *Gender & Psychoanal.*, 1:45-73.

Moglie, G. (1930), *Manuale di psichiatria* [*Handbook of Psychiatry*]. Roma: Luigi Pozzi Editore.

Montanari, M. (1996), *Psichiatria e psicopatologia dinamica* [*Dynamic Psychiatry and Psychopathology*]. Bologna: CLUEB.

Montano, A. (2000), *Psicoterapia con clienti omosessuali* [*Psychotherapy with Homosexual Clients*]. Milano: McGraw Hill.

Moor, P. (1985), *Omosessualità e Psicoanalisi* [Homosexuality and Psychoanalysis]. *Psicoterapia e Scienze Umane*, 19(4):48-58.

Moor, P. (1989), *Una ipocrisia psicoanalitica* [A psychoanalytic hypocrisy]. *Psicoterapia e Scienze Umane*, 23(2):61-68.

Morgenthaler, F. (1982), *L'omosessualità* [Homosexuality]. *Psicoterapia e Scienze Umane*, 16(4):3-39.

Morselli, A. (1915), *Manuale di psichiatria* [*Handbook of Psychiatry*]. Napoli: Idelson.

Musatti, C. (1949), *Trattato di psicoanalisi* [*Handbook of Psychoanalysis*]. Torino: Boringhieri.

Nobili, D. (1983), *L'omosessuale come capro espiatorio* [The homosexual as scapegoat]. *Rivista Sperimentale di Freniatria*, 107:117-128.

Oliverio Ferraris, A. (1994), *Omosessualità* [Homosexuality]. *Psicologia Contemporanea*, 126:22-31.

Pancheri, P. & Cassano, P. (1992), *Trattato italiano di psichiatria* [*Italian Textbook of Psychiatry*]. Milano: Masson.

Pancheri, P. & Cassano, P. (1999), *Trattato italiano di psichiatria* [*Italian Textbook of Psychiatry*]. Milano: Masson.

Passi Tognazzo, D. & Baratella, G. (1981), *I contenuti umani alle tavole III e IV del Rorschach in un gruppo di omosessuali maschi dell'Italia settentrionale* [Human contents in Rorschach Tables III and IV in a group of male homosexuals from Northern Italy]. *Rivista di psichiatria generale e dell'età evolutiva*, 19(1):1-7.

Pavanello Accerboni, A.M. (1984), *Il 'mito personale' di Umberto Saba tra poesia e psicoanalisi* [Umberto Saba's 'personal myth' between poetry and psychoanalysis]. *Rivista di Psicoanalisi*, 30,(4):546-559.

Penati, G. (1994), *Elementi di clinica e terapia psichiatrica* [*Elements of Psychiatric Practice and Therapy*]. Milano: Unicopli.

Petrella, F. (1992), *Esplorazioni nelle città di pianura: l'omosessuale in analisi* [Explorations in the cities of the plain: The homosexual in analysis]. *Rivista di Psicoanalisi*, XXXVIII(4):900-941.

Peyrefitte, R. (1949), *Les Amours singuliéres*. Italian Translation: *Eccentrici amori* [*Eccentric Loves*]. Milano: Longanesi, 1967.

Pietrantoni, L. (1999), *L'offesa peggiore* [*The Worst Offense*]. Pisa: Del Cerro Edizioni.

Reda, G.C. (1993), *Psichiatria, problemi, fenomeni, ipotesi, interventi* [*Psychiatry, problems, phenomena, hypotheses, interventions*]. Torino: UTET.

Rigliano, P. (2001), *Amore senza scandalo* [Love without Scandal]. Milano: Feltrinelli.

Romero, A. (1971), *L'infelice che ama la propria immagine* [The unhappy one who adores his own image: A problem of burning relevance]. *La Stampa*, April 15.

Rossi Barilli, G. (1999), *Il movimento gay in Italia* [*The Gay Movement in Italy*]. Milano: Feltrinelli.

Roughton, R. (1995), Overcoming antihomosexual bias: A progress report. *Amer. Psychoanalyst*, 29(4):15-16.

Roughton, R. (2001), Homosexuality: Clinical and technical issues. *Newsletter of the International Psychoanalytic Association*, 10(1):17-19.

Rubinstein, L.H. & Lopez, D. (1964), *Note sulla psicopatologia della prostituzione omosessuale* [Notes on the psychopathology of homosexual prostitution]. *Rivista Italiana di Psicoanalisi*, X(1):57-80.

Sarteschi, P. & Maggini, C. (1989), *Manuale di psichiatria* [*Handbook of Psychiatry*]. Bologna: SBM.

Savoia, V. (1998), *Omosessualità: un termine troppo vago e riduttivo ad un tempo* [Homosexuality: A term too vague and at the same time too reductive]. *Rivista di Psicoanalisi*, XLIV(2):331-336.

Schellenbaum, P. (1991), *Tra uomini. La dinamica omosessuale nella psiche maschile* [*Between Men: Homosexual Dynamics in the Male Psyche*]. Como: RED Edizioni, 1993.

Scoppa, A. (1978), *Medicina psichiatrica* [*Psychiatic Medicine*]. Napoli: Idelson.

Semi, A. ed. (1989), *Trattato di psicoanalisi* [*Textbook of Psychoanalysis*]. Milano: Raffaello Cortina.

Servadio, E. (1932), *Forme larvate di omosessualità* [Hidden forms of homosexuality]. *Rivista Italiana di psicoanalisi*, I(4):248-252.

Servadio, E. (1953), *Recenti vedute psicoanalitiche sulla genesi dell'omosessualità* [Recent psychoanalytic views on the origins of homosexuality]. *Ulisse*, 3(18):666-670.

Spaçal, S. (1982), *Il contributo psicoanalitico di Edoardo Weiss* [Edoardo Weiss's psychoanalytical contribution]. *Rivista di Psicoanalisi*, 28(1):97-118.

Tedeschi, G. (1953), *L'omosessualità e la psicoanalisi* [Homosexuality and psychoanalysis]. *Ulisse*, 3(18):637-665.

Vella, G. (1994), *Psichiatria e psicopatologia* [*Psychiatry and Psychopathology*]. Napoli: Idelson.

Walker, M. (1991), Jung and Homophobia. *Spring*, 51:55-69.

Weinberg, G. (1972), *Society and the Healthy Homosexual*. New York: Anchor Books.

Zucconi, C. (1983), *Omosessualità e pregiudizio* [Homosexuality and prejudice]. *Gli Argonauti*, 18:201-215.

From *"Long Yang"* and *"Dui Shi"*
to Tongzhi:
Homosexuality in China

Jin Wu, MA

SUMMARY. Homosexuality was widespread, recognized and fairly tolerated, although not entirely accepted, in ancient China. After being invaded and defeated by the Western powers in the mid- to late nineteenth century, "progressive" Chinese intellectuals at the turn of the twentieth century believed that Chinese traditions were "backward" and the actual cause of China's defeat; they looked to Westernization as a cure for the nation. This occurred at a time when homosexuality was regarded as a psychiatric condition in the West. Consequently, a pathological view of homosexuality and other antihomosexual attitudes were adopted by the Chinese along with Western technology and other "progressive thoughts." It was only after 1949 that homosexual behavior was seriously punished in China and served as grounds for persecution during Chinese political upheavals between the 1950s and 1970s. In the 1980s, the Chinese government's "open door" policy made it possible for the Chinese gay and lesbian community to develop; its bumpy journey since then reflected the fluctuation of the general political situation

---

Jin Wu is Social Worker and Child Specialist, Child Development Center of the Chinese American Service League (CASL), Chicago, IL.

In Chinese, the family name comes first and the given name comes last–the opposite of the order in English. In this paper, all Chinese names will appear in the Chinese order of family and given names. However, as the author has lived in the United States for over 10 years, he uses the English order for his own name: Jin (given name) Wu (family name).

[Haworth co-indexing entry note]: "From '*Long Yang*' and '*Dui Shi*' to Tongzhi: Homosexuality in China." Wu, Jin. Co-published simultaneously in *Journal of Gay & Lesbian Psychotherapy* (The Haworth Medical Press, an imprint of The Haworth Press, Inc.) Vol. 7, No. 1/2, 2003, pp. 117-143; and: *The Mental Health Professions and Homosexuality: International Perspectives* (ed: Vittorio Lingiardi, and Jack Drescher) The Haworth Medical Press, an imprint of The Haworth Press, Inc., 2003, pp. 117-143. Single or multiple copies of this article are available for a fee from The Haworth Document Delivery Service [1-800-HAWORTH. 9:00 a.m. - 5:00 p.m. (EST). E-mail address: getinfo@haworthpressinc.com].

10.1300/J236v07n01_08

in China over the last two decades. Despite the official pathologizing position of Chinese psychiatry–the prevailing view until recently–starting in the late 1980s, gay-friendly scholars and health professionals began to sympathetically research gay (*tongzhi*) communities in China and to advocate for sexual minorities. In 2001, the latest edition of the Chinese Classification of Mental Disorders (CCMD-3) removed the diagnosis of homosexuality per se but still retained a diagnosis resembling egodystonic homosexuality. Nevertheless, the *tongzhi* community in China has much work left to do before achieving full civil rights. *[Article copies available for a fee from The Haworth Document Delivery Service: 1-800-HAWORTH. E-mail address: <getinfo@haworthpressinc.com> Website: <http://www.HaworthPress.com> © 2003 by The Haworth Press, Inc. All rights reserved.]*

KEYWORDS. Ancient China, Chinese psychiatry, diagnostic categories, homosexuality, lesbianism, mental health professionals, *tongzhi*

THE ANCIENT TIME

In general, the ancient Chinese had rather open and accepting views of human sexuality until the 13th century. Today, many historical references available indicate that homosexuality was wide-spread, recognized and fairly tolerated, although not fully accepted, in ancient China (Ruan, 1991; Samshasha, 1997; Chou, 1997). In the last 20 years, gay activists and sympathetic scholars have presented such materials to challenge a modern, mainstream belief that previous societies in China did not have homosexuality and that it was "imported" from the West. Nevertheless, analysis of historical references has revealed that in ancient China, homosexuality was far from being fully accepted–although, unlike in Europe, in ancient China people were not seriously persecuted for engaging in same-sex sexual behavior (Samshasha, 1997).

In addition, in ancient China, there was no concept equivalent to a "gay" or "lesbian" identity; terms equivalent to the adjective "homosexual" were used to describe people's sexual behavior or a type of romantic relationship.[1] In ancient China, "homosexual" was only an adjective, never a noun (Chou, 1997). Same-sex encounters were only seen as behavior, not the core or some special nature of the person. There was no such concept as a "homosexual person." A person might engage in sexual relationships with a member of the other sex or with a person of the same sex. In any event, it was important for a man to get married and have legitimate offspring to continue the family line. Once that requirement was fulfilled, other sexual encounters could be tolerated; for example, wives' homosexual behavior in polygamous families could be an integrated part of family sexual life with the husband at the center (Ruan, 1991). Also, when the young male lovers of upper class men reached adulthood, their "masters" would help them marry women (Samshasha, 1997). Being married was a matter of social status.[2]

Furthermore, in ancient China, there was little questioning about the "cause" of homosexuality. Ruan (1991) reports a few speculations in ancient China on the causes of homosexuality, citing both "nature" and "nurture" as beliefs. However, none of these speculations occurred before the Ming Dynasty (1368-1644 A.D.), a time when the public attitudes of the Chinese people toward human sexuality were beginning to become more inhibited.

Male Homosexuality

Since only the activities of upper classes were recorded, there is little direct evidence in the historical records about homosexuality among common people in Ancient China, although some evidence can be found of its existence in fictional literature. Both Ruan Fang Fu's *Sex in China* (1991) and Samshasha's *History of Homosexuality in China* (1997) (the latter is available only in Chinese) give vast detailed accounts and citations of such works.

In *Sex in China* (1991), the famous Chinese sexologist Ruan Fang Fu states: "Male homosexuality may have been a familiar feature of Chinese life in prehistoric times. . . . China's earliest historical records contain accounts of male homosexuality" (p. 107). The ancient Chinese called men who had same-sex attraction *Long Yang* or *Xiang Gong*, and used terms like *yu tao* ("sharing the remaining peach") or *duan xiu* ("cut sleeve") to denote gay relationships.[3] Most of these names are based on allegorical tales which are briefly summarized below.

"*Yu Tao*" is the story of the love relationship between the king of Wei named Ling (534-493 B.C.) and his male lover Mi Tzu-hsia. One day, when wandering in the king's garden, Mi found an unusually sweet peach. After tasting it, he saved the remaining half and rushed back to the king, giving it to him. In Chinese, peach is pronounced "*tao*," and remaining is pronounced "*yu*," so "*yu tao*" can be translated as "sharing the remaining peach."

The lord, Long Yang, was a favorite male lover of another king, also in the state of Wei, several hundred years later. One day, while fishing with the king, Long Yang suddenly burst into tears. The king asked him why, and he replied that he was afraid that the king might give him up if he found more beautiful men, just as the king had considered giving up the smaller fish he had just caught. The king reassured him that would never happen, and issued an order that no one would be allowed to mention a more beautiful man in the presence of the king; if they did, the person's entire family would be executed. Later, Long Yang's name became a synonym for male homosexual love.

The *History of the (former) Han Dynasty (206 B.C.-A.D. 23) (Han Shu)* contained a special section describing the emperors' male sexual partners.[4] Ten out of the 11 emperors of the West Han Dynasty had at least one male lover or expressed attraction to men (Ruan, 1991). "Duan xiu" is the story of Han Ai-ti (who reigned from 6 B.C. to 1 A.D.) and his male lover, Dong Xian. One day, after taking a nap together, the emperor woke up before Dong. He found that the long sleeve of his robe was under Dong's body. Instead of waking him, the emperor decided to have the sleeve cut in order to avoid disturbing his lover. Thus "cut sleeve" came to refer to a homosexual relationship.

The term "Xiang Gong" originally meant "Your Excellency," "young master of a noble house," or "handsome young man" (Ruan, 1991, p. 115). In the Qing Dynasty, it was also used to refer to male actors who played female roles, and later came to mean the male lover of a man.[5] In the Qing Dynasty capital of Beijing, establishments known as *Xiang Gong Tang Zi* flourished. There, "feminine" men served male clients sexually. These businesses were abolished toward the end of the Qing dynasty and the beginning of the Republic, which was founded in 1912.[6]

Lesbianism

Although there are fewer accounts of lesbianism in ancient China, it was also tolerated, partly because the ancient Chinese believed that the women's supply of *Yin* (the substance and/or energy which is essential for the body) was unlimited in quantity (Ruan, 1991). Samshasha (1997) reports that some Western sinologists believe the attitude toward lesbianism in ancient China was more stable than that of male homosexuality, the status of which changed from dynasty to dynasty depending on the perferences of emperors and social atmospheres. The earliest mention of a lesbian relationship in the official historical record may be "*dui shi*" (*dui* can mean "facing each other," and *shi* means "eating, having a meal"). These were relationships between maids in the imperial court. In some couples, one would dress as a man and the other dressed as a woman and they called each other husband and wife. They ate and slept together. In the Ming and Qing Dynasties, there were erotic paintings which depicted merchants secretly selling sexual toys to maids in the imperial court with which they could enjoy each other sexually. There were also accounts in official and unofficial historical records of queens who were punished by the emperors after they were found sleeping with maids, even though some of these emperors had male concubines themselves. From the Tang Dynasty (617-907 AD) onward, there were also stories about sexual relationships between buddhist and taoist nuns. Ruan (1991) writes that lesbianism was considered inevitable and tolerated in some polygamous families, and sometimes even encouraged. An ancient sex handbook "give instructions for a method that not only allowed a man to enjoy two women at once, but simultaneously permitted pleasurable genital contact between the women" (p. 135).

The term *mojingzi* (rubbing mirrors or mirror grinding) is one of the traditional terms used to describe lesbian sexual behavior. Ruan (1991) reported that some formal associations of lesbians were found in the early period of the modern China. One of them, *Mojing Dang* ("Rubbing-mirrors Party"), was active in Shanghai in the late 19th century. "It was said to be a descendant of the 'Ten Sisters,' which a Buddhist nun had founded several hundred years earlier in Chaozhou, Guangdong (Canton) province. Members of the 'Ten Sisters' lived together as couples. They refused to marry, and some even avoided marriage by committing suicide" (p. 136). There were other names for relationships similar to the "ten sisters," including *"jin lan hui"* (golden orchid association), *"jin lan qi"* (golden orchid contact), *"shou pa jiao"* (handkerchief relationship), etc. Samshasha (1997) gives detailed accounts of *"jin lan hui"* between unmarried women who would raise silkworms to support themselves.[7] Some of these women turned their plait (the hairdo of an unmarried maid) into a bun (the hairdo of a married woman) and performed some ritual in the temple to formally announce their decision not to marry. Upon doing so, a woman's fiancee was not allowed to force the woman to marry, although his family could request her family to return the dowry. The two women would then share the cost for reimbursing the dowry. It might be presumptuous to assume that all of these women were lesbians, but some of them might have been.[8]

Today, modern scholars tend to believe that the acceptance of homosexuality was rooted in the traditional Chinese belief that a person's sex or gender is not fixed, rather relatively fluid, as is believed in many other non-Christian cultures (Samshasha, 1997; Chou, 1997). It was social class that defined a person's status. An upper class male's penis could enter a woman (who was in a lower class than a man), and other "lower-class" men. In *History of Homosexuality in China* (1997), Samshasha calls this feature of the Chinese culture "pansexualism" and "fuzzy transgender-transsexualism" (p. 12).

Antihomosexual Attitudes

Homosexuality, however, was not totally accepted in ancient China. Samshasha (1997) summarizes some examples of covert and overt antihomosexual attitudes in ancient China. Some are included below:

1. *Low social status of male sexual servants:* throughout the dynasties, male entertainers, who also served as male prostitutes for upper class men, were officially banned from taking official-select exams. These exams were a major means for people to advance their social status.

Anyone daring to falsify his identity to take such tests–and who passed–if found out could be killed or in any event immediately removed from their position and publicly humiliated.

2. *Revelation of same-sex attraction could ruin a career:* talented officials or writers could be punished if their attraction to or relationship with other men became known. For example, in South and North Dynasty (420-581 A.C.), a famous poet was removed from his government position after writing love letters to his male lover. Gay novels from the Ming Dynasty (1368-1644 A.C.) tell stories about students who were expelled from school for having same-sex romantic relationships.

3. *Derogatory and degrading descriptions of people engaged in same-sex sexual behavior:* in both official and unofficial historical records, as well as fictional literature works, there exist denigrating expressions used to describe same-sex attraction and romantic relationships.

In any event, compared to medieval Europe, homosexuality in ancient China was treated much more mildly. There was never any serious persecution for homosexual behavior alone.

EAST MEETS WEST:
THE INTRODUCTION OF PSYCHOLOGY
AND PSYCHIATRY INTO CHINA

After losing the Opium War in 1840 and most of the of wars in the ensuing decade fought by the Western powers on Chinese soil, China was forced to sign humiliating treaties, ceding Hong Kong and Macao and parts of major cities like Shanghai and Tianjing, and opened coastal cities along the Yangzi River as ports for international trade. "Semi-colonized" by the Western powers, the Chinese were not even permitted to stop the British from selling opium in China. For the first time in their history, the Chinese people experienced a serious threat from another part of the world. Defeated by Western technology, several generations of Chinese launched a series of "Westernization Movements." In the late nineteenth century, it was said: let "Chinese doctrine be the foundation and Western knowledge be the tool." This progressed to the "wholesale westernization" of the early twentieth century (Chou, 1997). However, this was a time when the dominant scientific approach in the West was positivism, and homosexuality was considered a mental disorder (Chou, 1997). Consequently, until the 1920s, "progressive" Chinese intellectuals viewed the traditional tolerance of homosexuality as backward as the Chinese traditions of forcing women to bind their feet, polygamy, pre-arranged marriage, and smoking opium. The "Colloquialism Movement" called for using everyday language to replace the hard-to-understand written language of antiquity. Although this vastly helped in improving literacy in China, it also made it difficult for people to access the historical records. As a result, the existence of homosexuality in ancient China became almost totally unknown after several generations (Samshasha, 1997; Chou, 1997).[9]

For example, the modern Chinese term for "homosexual(ity)" is composed of three characters: *tong* (the same) *xing* (sex, sexual, sexuality) and *lian* (attachment, romantic love, attraction). The term was coined around the beginning of the 20th century. Samshasha (1997) believes that it was probably derived from a Japanese translation of the German term, while Chou (1997) speculates that bilingual scholars, such as Yan Fu, might have been created it. In any event, in contrast to the terms used in ancient China, this term appears to have been adopted as part of the Westernization efforts.

Although psychological ideas can be found in Chinese writings dating back thousands of years (Gao et al., 1985; Lee and Petzold, 1987), traditional Chinese medicine is based on holistic perspectives. The mind-body connection is organically embedded in its principles and practice. Therefore, Chinese medicine did not need a specific specialty to take care of the mind as separated from the body. Modern Western psychology and psychiatry were introduced into China in the late nineteenth century. The first Chinese introduced to Western psychology were students sent by the imperial government to study in the West in the late 19th century. The Chinese Psychological Society was established in 1921 (Gao et al., 1985; Lee and Petzold, 1987). Lee and Petzold (1987) estimate that between 1922 and 1940, 370 books on psychology were published in China. Of these, over 40% were direct translations of texts from other countries, while the rest consisted mainly of textbooks based on Western materials and, to a lesser degree, research reports or monographs by Chinese psychologists. Most of the early leading psychologists in China were trained in the United States, with a handful coming from Great Britain and Germany.

Psychiatry as a specialty of Western medicine developed much later than other disciplines in China. Jon Kerr established the first modern psychiatric hospital in Guangzhou in 1897 (Thornicroft, 1988), but only a handful more of such institutions appeared in major cities in China over the next 50 years (Shen, 1993; Xia and Zhang, 1988.). Dr. Andrew Woods made the first attempt at psychiatric education in China while lecturing in Guangzhou in 1910, then in Beijing Union Medical College (PUMC) in 1919. Later, a few medical courses in major cities offered courses in psychiatry, although only irregularly. However, prior to 1949, there were no psychiatric professional organizations or journals in China and few people studied psychiatry (Xia and Zhang, 1988). As a profession, psychiatry had little impact on the lives of ordinary Chinese; most people with serious mental illness were either kept at home or became homeless (Thornicroft, 1988). Most people would seek help for family members suffering from mental illness from either traditional medicine practitioners or shamans.

Unsurprisingly, for both psychology and psychiatry in China, the initial period of development was dominated by Western schools of thought. These included Wundtian psychology, structuralism, functionalism, behaviorism, psychoanalysis and Gestalt psychology. As each school was introduced, each seemed to flourish, with different schools having greater influence in different parts of China (Lee and Petzold, 1987; Xia and Zhang, 1988). The Western concept of "mental health" was adopted in China in the 1930s and a few courses on the subject were offered in a handful of universities. The Chinese Mental Health Society was founded in 1936, but it had done little work by the time of its first regional conference in Nanjing in 1948 (Chen and Li, 1992). There is little reference to formal psychotherapy in China at that time (Zhong, 1991; Qian, 1994).

1949 TO THE LATE SEVENTIES: HOMOSEXUALITY IN CHINA DURING THE DARK AGES

After 1949, and for almost three decades, information from the West was almost completely unavailable in Mainland China. The changes and improvements in gay rights that were occurring in other parts of the world from the 1950s to the 1970s, or any information about gay life outside China, were rarely reported (Ruan, 1991). The few reports on gay life in the outside world were primarily used as examples of the "decline and evil of Western civilization" (p. 121). These conditions created a sense of isolation for gays and lesbians in China. Nonetheless, homosexual behavior had never disappeared in China.

Arguably, this was the most sexually repressive period in the history of China. During this time, homosexual behavior could be grounds for persecution. Punishment ranged from labor under surveillance to imprisonment for years, depending upon the political atmosphere at the time and the mood of the specific authorities. After the end of the Cultural Revolution in late 1970s, as the government spent several years "rehabilitating" people who had been persecuted, those persecuted due to same-sex behaviors did not receive the same treatment (Wan, personal communication, 1997, 2001).

In fact, there have never been any mention in the criminal laws of the People's Republic of China (PRC) which specifically address homosexual behavior. An umbrella term, "hooliganism," which was dropped from the penal code in 1997, covered a wide range of behaviors which included extra-marital and pre-marital sexual behaviors, sodomy and other "socially indecent" and "sexually promiscuous" behaviors, as well as minor sexual assault. The sentence for hooliganism could range from several days of detention up to 7 years of imprisonment. An adult who engaged in sodomy with a minor could be sentenced from 7 years to life imprisonment (Zhang, 1994).

After 1949, China was strongly influenced by the Soviet Union until the break-up of the Sino-Soviet relationship in the late 1950s. During that time, Soviet theories were adopted while Western schools of thoughts were criticized and abolished (Gao et al., 1985; Li, Xu and Kuang, 1988). "Learning from the Soviet Union completely" was the most influential slogan in the early 1950s in China (Zhang, 1988).[10] Academics and professionals underwent "thought reform" (Ding, 1991). Marxism and Pavlov's high nervous activity theory became the official guideline for psychology in China. Soviet textbooks were translated into Chinese and adopted as textbooks in China.[11]

The role official psychiatry played in political persecution was very different in the Soviet Union and China. As is now widely known, during the Stalin era and later, political dissidents were labeled as mentally ill and locked up in psychiatric hospitals. During China's Cultural Revolution (1966-1976), mental disorders were seen as the result of either immorality or "backward thoughts." Psychiatric patients were put in "study groups," required to read newspapers or given lectures on "correct thoughts."

At that time in China, only severe mental conditions such as psychosis and mental retardation were considered to be mental disorders, as well as a generic term *shen jing shuai ruo* which referred to neuroses. Although homosexual behavior was seen as a sexual disorder, it was rarely treated psychiatrically. It was mainly dealt with as a criminal behavior or as a bad habit. The small number of psychiatrists who did treat "homosexuals" between the 1950s and 1970s believed homosexuality was a "thought problem" or a political stand which could be corrected with class-education and labor reform (Chou, 1996).

THE 1980s: AFTER THE DOOR OPENED

In the early 1980s, the Chinese government adopted the "Open Door" policy. Information from outside China became more available and ordinary people started having more freedom. The Chinese gay and lesbian community rose under these conditions, although its bumpy journey reflects the fluctuation of the political atmosphere in China over the last two decades. The term *tongzhi* (see below) has been adopted as a name for the community of gay and lesbian people. Currently, the *tongzhi* communities are fairly visible in all major cities, and there are more than 250 Chinese *tongzhi* web sites in and outside China. However, the changes have mainly benefited people in large urban centers and in academic circles. The 1997 deletion of "hooliganism" from the penal code is considered to be the official decriminalization of homosexuality. Although the official position viewed homosexuality as a mental disorder until recently, the actual views of scholars and heath professionals have been some-what diverse for the last 20 years, and some research and advocacy work has been done in the last decade.

One of the direct consequences of the open door policy was that information from outside China flooded in, including information about human sexuality. Despite government attempts to "sweep away the yellow subjects"[12] in the mid-1980s, "a sex [sic] revolution appeared in China in 1986" (Pan, 1993, p. 59). A national survey conducted in 1989-1990 showed that 86% of people approved of premarital sex, while the government estimated, in the late 1980s, that about 30% of (heterosexual) couples living together had not registered le-gally (Ruan, 1991).

Throughout the 1980s, while gay and lesbian populations were becoming more visible in the West, in China, as a general rule, homosexuality was basi-cally unknown. Ruan (1991) quotes a story reported by Lenore Norrgard, a Se-attle-based freelance writer and an activist in 1990: ". . . two young women who went to the Marriage Bureau to register their bond, and were promptly ar-rested. . . . Homosexuality is illegal in China, yet ignorance about it is so vast that the two apparently were not even aware of the taboo" (p. 140). Richard Green, in his *Series Editor's Comment* on Ruan's *Sex in China* (1991) states that when he taught at Meijing Union Medical College (arguably the best med-ical school in China) in 1988, some of the physicians there told him there were no homosexuals in China.

The concept of bisexuality was even less known in China at that time. Most English-Chinese dictionaries published in China up to the mid-1980 defined the word "bisexual" as "having both sexes" or an "organism with both sexes in it," with no mention of its meaning as a sexual orientation. In a 1992 paper on the analysis of 1000 "homosexual" cases in the *Chinese Mental Health Jour-nal*, the authors called the attraction to both sexes "dual orientation" (Lu et al., 1992).

However, in the 1980s people started to learn about homosexuality as something which existed outside China. For example, people in urban centers, especially in academic circles, had access to Western literature; some of them might have met openly gay or lesbian Westerners.[13] Meanwhile, small com-munities of gay and lesbian people in various parts of China were quietly de-veloping.

THE OFFICIAL POSITION AND GOVERNMENT PRACTICE

As previously stated, after the Cultural Revolution, the illegal status of ho-mosexuality remained unchanged until 1997. In general, the policy was not used to arrest people engaged in homosexual behavior unless they were reported or found in public space. But, in reality, given the isolation and housing shortage, for many gay men, cruising sites were the only places they could find each other. However, once arrested, a person could be detained up to 15 days or sentenced to several-year forced labor or imprisonment, largely depending the political atmosphere at the time (Li and Wang, 1992; Wan, 1997). Police and neighborhood watchdogs often patrolled sites where gay men gathered (usually parks, public restrooms or bathhouses) and made arrests from time to time. Arrested gay men were subject to humiliation and even beatings, as well as charged with fines. In the early and mid-1990s, probably the police's motivation for arresting gay men had more to do with their economic gain (Wan, 1997). Sometimes arrested people were allowed to leave without pressing charges, sometimes their employers were notified and were asked to take them back (Zhang, 1994). Gay men would rather undergo any humiliation instead of being exposed to their families or employers. However, it varied how the employers dealt with the cases–from no punishment, to reduced salary or no pay for a limited time, to demotion, to firing (Li and Wang, 1992).

From the 1980s to the mid-1990s, the most common punishment for gay men was not legal, but administrative punishment within the workplace.[14] Administrative punishment ranged from demotion or losing pay for a period of time to being fired. This was at a time when the only available jobs were government-assigned. Such punishment also resulted in losing face in one's community, which is a major concern in Chinese culture. If exposed, gay men with higher social status could lose status, as well as current and potential income. However, they also had more protection. For example, a Communist Party member might lose his party membership, while a non-Party-member could go to jail for the same behavior (Li and Wang, 1992). One attitude of the government and police was that sexually receptive gay men (bottoms) were punished less harshly–sometimes even avoiding any punishment–than insertive gay men who "played the active roles" (tops) (Li and Wang, 1992). This may have to do with the authorities' conceptualization of sodomy–the penetrating partner was the perpetrator and the receiving one was the victim. Legal and administrative punishments for lesbians are not very common, but they are more vulnerable to social pressures (see below).

THE POSITIONS OF PSYCHIATRISTS AND OTHER SCHOLARS

In the late 1970s, the emphasis of psychiatry in China shifted from "thought reform" to a biological model which conceptualized mental disorders as being like other medical conditions. At that time, this was a natural and progressive reaction to the beliefs of the Cultural Revolution. It removed the blame from the patients and gave more room for the person to receive help. The bio-psycho-social model was introduced in the late '80s when most psychiatrists tended to see things from a traditional medical perspective.

The standard diagnostic tool in Chinese psychiatry was initially discussed in 1958 and the first version of the *Chinese Classification of Mental Disorders* (CCMD) was published in 1978 (Shen, 1993). Homosexuality was classified as a sexual disorder, regardless of the person's attitude toward his or her homosexual tendency. The CCMD-2 was published in 1989, and CCMD-2-R in 1994; both clearly stated that Chinese clinicians were not to accept the changing, non-pathological view of homosexuality emerging in other parts of the world (Chinese Psychiatric Association & the Neurological Hospital, Nanjing Medical University, 1995). Although the official statement did reflect the majority's view, opinions of people in the field were quite diverse, ranging from "crime" or "disorder," to "unclear" to "natural," even to "a matter of minority's oppression by a majority." Such viewpoints were also clearly reflected in most psychiatric textbooks and other publications at that time (Zhang, 1994).

Up to the early 1990s, the mainstream of Chinese psychiatry and the social sciences saw homosexuality as "a strange disease that deserves denunciation . . . a special mistake that is against human nature, an abnormal behavior that should be severely prohibited and punished, and a problem that apparently has something to do closely with morality" (Zhang, 1994, p. 576).[15] Some believed that homosexuality "threatens the social order, destroys the health of youth, and disturbs the harmony of other people's family" (p. 577). Some psychiatrists believed that gay people tended to sexually violate other people or could convert them to homosexuality. Some also believed that "homosexuals" could not maintain their well-being and productivity since homosexuality was "against the law of biology." Some even stated that AIDS was nature's punishment. Some psychiatrists supported the harsh punishments meted out to gay men in parts of China and said it was "understandable and necessary" (p. 577). Some held that homosexuality was caused by capitalist system and beliefs; some felt it necessary to criticize the "bourgeois liberalization" that was taking place in the 1980s as a necessary measure for preventing homosexuality in China. Some scholars strongly opposed any tolerance of homosexuality.

Although harsh about homosexuality as a phenomenon, many Chinese psychiatrists at that time also showed respect to and sympathy for gay people; some considered sexual orientation immutable, although they still viewed homosexuality as a disorder. Many scholars denounced discrimination against "homosexuals" and admitted that punishment would not help in preventing or eliminating homosexuality (Zhang, 1994). Some psychiatrists genuinely believed that the pathological label would protect gay people. Some said, "when the police arrest somebody for homosexual behavior, I testify that it is a disease. Then they release him. Simple as that" (Zhang Beichuan, personal communication, 1998).

In 1992, Lu et al. published a paper in the *Chinese Mental Health Journal* which analyzed 1000 "homosexual cases" accumulated over 10 years in psychiatric outpatient settings throughout the country. It is probably the largest sample of "homosexuals" studied in China up to that point[16] and still one of the largest to date.

The authors concluded that homosexuality was caused by poor discipline in childhood, a lack of male role models (although a small percentage of the sample were females) and dominant mothers. They insisted not to give up on treatment for "real homosexuals," and believed that more research on the cause of homosexuality would help in preventing it, which would vastly benefit society. However, in correspondence with one of the authors in 1998, I was told they had stopped trying to change people's sexual orientation; instead, they wanted to use their authority roles to help their gay clients accept themselves.

Some psychiatrists said that they had stopped using aversion therapy because it was inhumane. Others used a method called "desensitization," similar to guided imagery. Based on the belief that male "homosexuals" had difficulty being intimate with women, patients were asked to relax and imagine being with a young woman in a favorite place (Fang, 1995). In a 1999 survey of psychotherapists by Cong and Gao, respondents reported several therapy modalities that they used in working with "homosexuals," including cognitive therapy (40.0%), psychoanalysis (25.7%), eclectic therapy (20.0%), behavioral therapy (5.7%), supportive therapy (5.7%), and family system therapy (2.9%). There are anecdotal reports of individuals being treated with psychotropic medications to change their sexual orientation as well.

Non-pathologizing viewpoints within the psychiatric community, although a minority, were also expressed occasionally. In 1985, a leading sexologist Ruan Fang Fu,[17] using the pseudonym Hua Jin Ma, published an article in a popular magazine, *To Your Health.* He not only addressed the existence of same-sex attraction in many parts of the world and throughout the history of the human race, but also stated that pathologizing homosexuality was a matter of the majority's oppressing a minority. That was the first statement of this kind made publicly in Mainland China. Ruan's article received 60 letters from readers, including 56 from gay men from all over China. An analysis of the letters was published in *Archives of Sexual Behavior* in 1988.

THE RISE OF GAY AND LESBIAN COMMUNITIES

In late 1990, partly due to the AIDS threat, the Chinese government realized it had to deal with the gay population, which led to a series of unexpected events that contributed to the development of the LGB community in China over the next 10 years. The political mood in China affected the vicissitudes of that process. Health educator Wan Yan Hai of the Institute of Health Education, under the Health Ministry, was assigned to do the AIDS prevention work. He eventually turned his work into gay advocacy. In April 1992, he set up China's first AIDS hotline in Beijing. He and his hotline volunteers went to gay gathering places to distribute educational materials and gradually gained trust from them (Fang, 1995). Then in November 1992, he hosted the first gay men club, "Men's World," in Beijing. It offered monthly gatherings for gay men for free discussion. Initially, his work was supported by the government and widely reported in the media both in and outside China (Wan, 1997). However, in late 1993, the political atmosphere changed. Wan was ordered to stop his advocacy work and Men's World was closed down. Refusing to comply, Wan was fired from his job in 1994, and his supportive superior was demoted.

Following that, Wan became a freelance writer and educator and started his AIDS Action Project, continuing his AIDS education and gay advocacy work. He published a newsletter, the *AIZHI* Newsletter, with information on gay and lesbian rights and life, sexual education and AIDS prevention materials, as well as related research both in and outside China. He distributed the newsletter free of charge to scholars, government officials, educators, gay men and lesbians, as well as the general public. He hosted workshops and offered lectures on gay rights and AIDS prevention in Beijing whenever possible, and worked with numerous individual gay men, lesbians and people with HIV or AIDS in different parts of China.

In the early 1990s, gay activists from Hong Kong and Taiwan began to go to China to research and help build the community. In the mid and late 1990s, Hong Kong sociologist Chou Wah Shan stayed in China at length and published, both as author and editor, a number of books on the situations for sexual minorities in China from different angles (Chou, 1996, 1997; Wu and Chou, 1996). Hong Kong activist and publisher John Loo also traveled to China many times, and published gay and lesbian fictional writings by authors from Hong Kong, Taiwan, and Mainland China (Loo, 1996; 1999; Cui, 1997).

Activists from Hong Kong and Taiwan also brought into China a new term for the LGB community, *tongzhi*, the Chinese equivalent of "comrade."[18] This usage was coined by Hong Kong gay activist Mike in 1987, as a way to translate the term "gay and lesbian" for the 1988 Hong Kong Gay and Lesbian Movie Festival (Chou, 1997). Widely used by LGB communities in Hong Kong, Taiwan, and southeast Asian countries with large Chinese populations, the term was introduced into China in the mid-1990s. At that time of its introduction into China, the gay and lesbian communities had few terms to describe themselves. Ancient terms like *long yang* and *duan xiu* (see above) were unknown to young people. The technical term, "*tong xing lian*," is too formal and carries negative, even shameful connotations; it had been widely used by psychiatrists to describe a mental disorder, so the gay and lesbian community did not want to use it. *Tongzhi* filled in a blank.[19]

Despite some setbacks, 1994 continued to see some media coverage of gay-related issues, including a few coming out stories (Wan Yan Hai, personal communication, 1995). Several monographs on homosexuality were published around that time, something which had not happened since 1949. Although homophobic by today's standards, all of the authors claimed that homosexuality was normal and that they were trying to raise people's consciousness on the matter. All of those authors experienced difficulty finding publishers.[20]

In December, 1994, a symposium on AIDS and sex education took place in Beijing, hosted by the famous bioethicist Qiu Ren Zong at the Chinese Academy of Social Science. Approximately 50 scholars and other participants reached a 12-point consensus, accepting homosexuality as a normal phenomenon and urging more communication and understanding between different sectors of society. Encouraged by the success of the symposium, the organizers decided to hold a similar meeting in early 1996, mainly for gay and lesbian people. About 70 people registered, and funds were raised, both within and outside China, to subsidize the participation of low-income people. However, at the last minute, the public security department ordered the meeting postponed and it never took place. Nevertheless, the organizers managed to collect papers from the potential participants; the effort to publish them resulted in the establishment of the *Friends* newsletter in early 1998, published by Zhang Beichuan and his colleagues at the Qingdao Medical College and other institutions.[21]

Tongzhi communities were also developing among overseas Mainland Chinese citizens, mostly students, as a way to end isolation and support each other. Most of such groups were primarily social in nature. In 1997, Wan Yan Hai, Lin Eryan and I, along with some other Chinese students and visiting scholars in North America, founded the Chinese Society for the Study of Sexual Minorities (CSSSM). Its mission was to disseminate updated information on homosexuality and gay rights to the *tongzhi* community and the general public in China, and to enlist support in depathologizing homosexuality in China. One of the main project carried out by the CSSSM is its biweekly, bilingual webzine *tao hong man tian xia* (pink color all over the world), written primarily in Chinese with some news summaries in English.[22] The 1997 revision of the penal code was a significant milestone for the *tongzhi* community.[23] In June 1998, Chinese gay activist Gary Wu organized the first Chinese *tongzhi* conference in North America in San Francisco. About 150 Chinese *tongzhi* participated, including some from Hong Kong, Taiwan, Japan, and other countries.

In October 1998, the first lesbian conference in China took place in Beijing; more then 30 women from all over the country attended. As a result, *Beijing Sister*, a lesbian activist group, was formed. The first lesbian web site in China had been set up in August of that year, and several more appeared soon after. In November 1998, an open lesbian participated in a symposium on feminism hosted by the Chinese Academy of Social Science. Her dialogue with feminist scholars resulted in a panel discussion by lesbians in the following year's similar symposium. In December 1998, the first delegate from China attended the conference of the Asian Lesbian Network in Manila. In 1999, a lesbian delegate from China attended an international gay and lesbian conference in South Africa. A connection between the Chinese *tongzhi* community and the international LGBT communities had been established.

Media exposure about gay issues reached a new level on December 20, 2000. Openly gay and lesbian people appeared on TV in China for the first time on Hunan province TV station's talk show, "Let's Talk." Its last episode in the twentieth century was on the topic of homosexuality. Guests included an openly gay male professor and writer, an openly lesbian artist, and sociologist Li Yin He, one of the top scholars in China who has studied gay subculture. More than a dozen people from the audience asked various questions, and expressed their opinions which ranged from opposing homosexuality to viewing it as natural phenomenon. Such an open and friendly discussion would not be imaginable just a few years ago (Hunan TV, 2000).

In 2001, the three major events in the *tongzhi* community were the lesbian cultural festival in May, the conference on *tongzhi* web sites and AIDS education in November, and the *tongzhi* movie festival at Beijing University in December. The lesbian cultural festival was stopped by the police just before it began. The *tongzhi* movie festival started well and received vast media coverage, but it was ordered to stop early. Only the conference on *tongzhi* web sites and AIDS education took place smoothly.[24]

Nevertheless, in major cities in China, gay and lesbian gatherings are becoming commonplace and commercial gay bars also exist in all big cities. For example, in Beijing, gay men who participate in some community activities are numbered in the thousands; lesbians in the hundreds. However, these number are a small fraction of the gay and lesbian populations in the city. The majority of people in China attracted to people of the same sex are still isolated. Even in the active gay and lesbian communities, people still have to be very cautious. The common practice in those communities is not to disclose real names, occupations, employers, etc. It is obviously difficult to maintain long-term gay or lesbian relationships in this climate. However, cyberspace can compensate for some of the inconvenience of the physical world. The Internet and the World Wide Web have developed rapidly in China in the last few years, and the *tongzhi* communities have found this new territory especially useful.[25]

Nonetheless, *tongzhi* websites, like other websites in China, may face government censorship. If its content is considered pornographic or too critical of the government, a website hosted within China could be warned or even closed down. A website hosted outside China might be blocked and made inaccessible from within China.

It should also be pointed out that although some young people adopt the identities of gay, lesbian or bisexual, the majority of people in China attracted to people of the same sex do not see their sexual orientations as their primary identities. Many of them are married and raise their families. Western readers should not attribute this as only being due to their not having other choices. Although a lack of choices is definitely part of the reason, a cultural tradition that emphasizes social status and family relations plays an important role, too.

BECOMING NORMAL: A NEW BEGINNING

The third edition of the Chinese Classification of Mental Disorders (CCMD-III)–passed by the Chinese Psychiatric Association at the end of 2000, and published in April 2001–dropped the diagnosis of homosexuality per se but added a diagnosis of ego-dystonic homosexuality. Considering that in the late 1990s the majority of psychiatrists in China still supported pathologizing homosexuality, this change is quite remarkable (Cong and Gao, 1999; Wan, 2001). As the following account illustrates, it is also the result of efforts by both *tongzhi* activists and psychiatrists.

In September 1996, the Chinese Psychiatric Association (CPA) formed a task force to revise the CCMD-II-R and produce the CCMD-III. For the first time, the *tongzhi* community responded in a united way. The AIZHI Action Project soon proposed to depathologize homosexuality in China (Wan, 2001). From October to December of that year, Wan Yan Hai and his colleagues embarked upon a number of projects. They conducted telephone interviews with some of the task force members to ask for their opinions on homosexuality; they searched for and contacted gay-friendly psychiatrists and urged them to participate in the deletion of homosexuality from CCMD. Wan edited a special issue of the AIZHI Newsletter which included information on the current situation of homosexuality in the world, the American Psychological Association's Policy Statements on Gay, Lesbian and Bisexual Issues, and other materials related to civil rights and minority rights issues. The newsletter was mailed to all CCMD task force members, some 170 psychiatric hospitals, and almost 300 psychologists, sexologists and other heath care professionals nationwide (Wan, 2001).[26]

In January 1997, Wan came to the United States as a visiting scholar at Southern California University.[27] In February of that year, the idea of establishing the Chinese Society for the Study of Sexual Minorities (CSSSM) was put forward, and the group was formally founded that September.[28] A major focus of the CSSSM was to contact professional and activist organizations in the West to enlist support for the deletion of homosexuality from the CCMD in particular, and for the development of the *tongzhi* community in China in general. In regard to the CCMD, information was shared in professional conferences, newsletters and list serves. Due to the CSSSM's efforts, in 1998, both the American Psychological Association and the American Psychiatric Association wrote letters to the Chinese Psychiatric Association in support of removing homosexuality from the CCMD-III. In March 1998, the American Counseling Association passed a resolution supporting the removal of homosexuality from the CCMD-III. In September 1998, the *APA Monitor* published an article reporting the revision of CCMD and the work of the CSSSM (Sleek, 1998). Also in 1998, the president of the American Psychiatric Association, Herbert Sacks, MD, at a joint conference with Chinese psychiatrists in Beijing, addressed the importance of deleting homosexuality from the list of mental disorders.

Within China, there was a discussion of the diagnostic status of homosexuality in *Zhejiang (Province) Mental Health Information*, a monthly newspaper published by the Mental Health Institute of Zhejiang Province and targeted to the general public. It has been called the "first open debate on homosexuality" in the media in China. From August 1997 to February 1998, a total of 11 articles were published, 4 of which supported depathologizing homosexuality[29] and five of which opposed depathologization;[30] the other two articles were ambiguous on whether homosexuality is a mental disorder but nevertheless considered homosexuality to be abnormal.[31] The Jia article which opened the debate illustrates Chinese psychiatry's anti-gay viewpoint then–and perhaps even now.[32] Jia listed three major "harmful effects" of homosexuality: disturbing societal harmony–including increased sexual crime, disintegrating families, and spreading STDs and AIDS. He regarded Americans who believed "AIDS is God's punishment of gays" as sensible people. He maintained that the majority of Chinese people would not agree to depathologizing homosexuality as it was contrary to the Chinese moral code and psychological principles. He insisted that any group composing less than 5% of the general population should be seen as deviant, and that since "homosexuals" composed a very small portion of the population in China, it would be reasonable and lawful to classify homosexuality as a sexual disorder.[33] He further went on to assert that the removal of homosexuality from the DSM-III and IV and from the ICD-10, was due to biases caused by social and political demands–and that China should set up a classification system with its own characteristics.

The Chinese Psychiatric Association's task force conducted a research project using "homosexuals" recruited primarily from the gay and lesbian community in Beijing (Wan, 2001), as well as some individuals who sought mental health services (Liu et al., 1999).[34] Activists praised the task force for going into the community, instead of only using subjects in the clinical population.[35] However, the tone of the report is ambiguous about whether homosexuality is normal. For example, in the discussion section, before stating that homosexuality per se is not a mental disorder, the report says: "Because homosexuality violates the law of biology, differing from the sexual orientation of the majority of human population, it was considered a mental disorder. Currently, it is still in debate if homosexuality should be an object of medical and psychiatric research and treatment" (Liu, 2001, p. 101, translation of author). The main findings and conclusions from the task force's report were:

- The cause of "homosexuality" is complex and "related to bio-psycho-social factors" (Liu, 2001, p. 89). Nevertheless, the researchers speculated that, given that some homosexual subjects grew up in families with disharmony or were raised by grandparents, a lack of "normal family atmosphere," particularly the love of fathers and mothers, could be part of the reason for an individual to become "homosexual."
- Using the EPQ and MMPI, one cannot distinguish "homosexual" people from heterosexuals; however, gay and lesbian subjects have high scores on some clinical scales of the MMPI, such as hypochondria, hysteria, schizophrenia, depression, and hypomania.
- The majority (44) of the subjects had sought mental health or other services to change their sexual orientation but none of them had succeeded in doing so.
- The researchers only identified 6 subjects who had ever needed clinical treatment, therefore concluded that the majority of "homosexuals" were not ill.
- One-third of the subjects had suicide attempts.[36]
- Homosexuality per se should not be considered a mental disorder, but "homosexuals" experiencing distress due to their sexual orientation need mental health services.

The ambivalence of the task force's report reflects overall attitudes of psychiatrists in China. The most recent data on the attitudes of mental health professionals in China toward homosexuality is that of Cong Zhong and Gao Wenfeng (1999) published in *Chinese Journal of Behavioral Medical Science*. In 1998, the authors surveyed 47 psychotherapists from all over the country who participated in a workshop that was part of a joint Chinese-German training series on psychoanalysis. The respondents showed some acceptance and tolerance toward gay people. The majority of the respondents (73.9%) believed homosexuality had nothing to do with morality; 17.4% said it was immoral. Almost two-thirds (65%) saw gay people as lawful citizens; 20% saw them as antisocial; 5% saw them as promiscuous, and 2.5% saw them as evil. When asked if homosexuality was legal in China, a year after "hooliganism" was removed from the criminal law, 54.5% said yes, 38.6% said no, and 6.8% said irrelevant.

In considering the question of whether homosexuality is normal, the picture changed somewhat: 56.5% of the respondents considered it "not a disorder but also not normal;" 17.4% considered it totally normal and 26.1% considered it a mental disorder. Regarding the removal of homosexuality from the upcoming edition of CCMD, overall, 48.6% of the respondents supported removal, while 51.4% opposed it. When the sample was broken down into two groups–psychologists and psychiatrists–about 2/3 of psychologists supported removal and about 2/3 of psychiatrists opposed it.

On average, each respondent had seen 7.5 "homosexual clients" in outpatient settings, with the highest number of 45. The majority of "homosexual clients" seen were gay men, with a small number of lesbians and bisexuals. The main reasons for seeking psychotherapy were social pressure (60.5%), difficulty in accepting oneself (44.2%), lack of understanding from family members (44.2%), homophobia (the authors did not specify) (41.9%), desire to change sexual orientation (32.6%), socialization and employment (30.2%), and being forced into heterosexual marriages (23.3%).

About half of the respondents believed the distress their "homosexual clients" suffered was due to a clients' own weaknesses, while others considered the distress to be caused by society. When asked how gay people's mental health compared with heterosexuals, 55% respondents thought it was poorer, 42.5% thought it the same, one respondent thought it better. Respondents believed the causes (more than one answer was allowed) of homosexuality included: postnatal psychological development and educational influence (93.0%), seduction by others (41.9%), genetic (37.2%), postnatal physical development (30.2%), social and cultural causes (18.6%), and other (11.6%). Psychotherapy modalities used with these clients included cognitive therapy (40.0%), psychoanalysis (25.7%), and eclectic therapy (20.0%). In ascertaining the therapists' main goals for their clients, the picture was mixed: self-acceptance (81.4%), adjustment (81.4%), and change of sexual orientation (30.2%). The effectiveness of psychotherapy reported 2.6% totally cured, 15.4% significantly improved, 64.1% improved, and 17.9% no change.[37]

CONCLUSION

The removal of homosexuality from the CCMD-III–widely reported in China and all over the world–stirred up much discussion in the *tongzhi* community. Many people welcomed the change, while some others criticized it for incompleteness (Wan, 2001). The actual status of homosexuality in China at this point is that it is "not a disorder but it is also not normal." The fate of the first gay and lesbian film festival provides an interesting footnote on the current state of affairs. The festival sponsored by the Movie Association at Peking University was planned for December 14 through 23, 2001. It was to show a number of gay and lesbian movies made in China, Taiwan and many Western countries. After the films were shown, it was to include a number of workshops led by renowned scholars on topics from gay and lesbian movies to global gay and lesbian movements (Leinng, 2001). However, around December 20, the authority of Peking University decided to cancel the workshops. As it turns out, some media agencies had not only reported on the festival, they also gave in-depth coverage on gay lives and homosexuality. It was this coverage which prompted Peking University officials to ask the Movie Association to cancel the workshops because "this activity sponsored by the Movie Association was suspected of 'using this opportunity to rectify the reputation of homosexuals'" (Scat09, 2001). Clearly, the *tongzhi* community in China has much work left to do before achieving full civil rights. However, simple imitation of the LGB world in the West may not be the solution for the *tongzhi* community in China. As Samshasha (1997) suggests, part of the answer may be indigenous and found in Chinese history.

NOTES

1. A note on word usage: In this paper, I mainly use "gay and lesbian" instead of "gay, lesbian and bisexual" for two reasons. First it is less wordy. This is not to say that bisexuality has not been discussed in the sexual minority community, nor is it a denial of any discrimination of bisexual people in the community. Second, and more importantly, mainstream thinking in China today, when focusing on a person's homosexuality, considers the "heterosexual" side to be simply "normal."

2. Samshasha (1997) also reports an even more ironic phenomenon: in the late Qing Dynasty, when the imperial government banned male prostitute brothels, many of the high officials who used to patronize them, suddenly started visiting female prostitutes! Samshasha speculated that those married upper class men might have seen same-sex sexual encounters as a safe way of seeking extra-marital sexual pleasure while avoiding extra-marital reproduction, which could bring long-term trouble for them.

3. Chronologically, the story of "yu tao" is the oldest–from the Spring and Autumn period of the Zhou Dynasty (779-476 B.C.), then "Long Yang," from the Warring States period of the Zhou Dynasty (475-221 B.C.), then "duan xiu" from the West Han Dynasty (206 B.C.-A.D. 23) (Ruan, 1991; Samshasha, 1997). The name "Xiang Gong" appeared much later, in the Qing Dynasty (A.C. 1644-1911) (Ruan, 1991).

4. This practice did not continue in the Later Han Dynasty or in any of the ensuing dynasties.

5. Among these well-known terms referring to male homosexuality, "Xiang Gong" is the only one which does not come from the upper class. Ruan (1991) believes that this term is similar to "drag queen" and "hustler," and could be translated as "she-male."

6. Male prostitution for men existed throughout the history of China and up to the late Qing Dynasty (Ruan, 1991). Even during the Republic, there were still a small number of male prostitutes in big cities like Shanghai who were subject to humiliation and rough treatment from the upper class men who hired them (Samshasha, 1997).

7. During the Qing Dynasty, beginning in the Shende area of Guangdong Province.

8. Some might have been attracted to men but simply refused to put themselves in a powerless position. Since heterosexual coupling was the only model of adult life in China, and since family relationships were so essential at that time, some of them might have simply wanted to form their living units in the same form to support each other.

9. Western Christian missionaries also contributed to reinforcing antihomosexual attitudes in China. The first Christian missionaries came to China during the late Ming Dynasty (late seventeenth century), but never gained much favor in the imperial court; some of the early ones were even killed by the Chinese. Early missionaries were astonished when they saw Chinese men holding hands and displaying affection in public. They saw this as evidence that the Chinese people were uncivilized and in need of salvation (Chou, 1997). After the Opium War, and defended by the Western power's military might, Christian missionaries had much more leeway to spread their beliefs which included the concept of homosexuality as sin (Chou, 1997).

10. As many in China criticized, at that time and decades later, that this was another attempt to look for a cure-all from an external source. The vast differences between the two cultures actually made such adoption not much deeper than the surface.

11. It is not entirely clear how the Soviet influence affected China on issues related to homosexuality. Homosexuality was officially, as well as practically, accepted in Soviet Union until the early 30s (Samshasha, 1997). Stalin reinstalled the Tsar's banning of sodomy, which must have been known in China in the 1950s. However, by then antihomosexual attitudes had already been prevailing in China for half a century.

12. "Yellow" in China, like "blue" in the US, means erotic or pornographic.

13. An American professor who is gay told me that, when he taught in Beijing in the early 1980s, his partner visited him in the summer. Their relationship was known to most of his students and Chinese colleges and they did not make it a big deal.

14. In China, especially when most people had to work for the government, "administrative punishement," including but not limited to being suspended without pay, salary cuts, demotion, and/or being fired, was considered a less severe punishment than a legal one. It is a part of the government control of the social order, applicable to everyone, not only to Communist Party members. Even the neighhood association has this kind of control over people who do not have jobs.

15. Statements from Zhang, 1994 are translated by Jin Wu.

16. The English translation of this paper, translated by Jin Wu and edited by A. R. D'Augelli, is available from the American Psychological Association, 750 First Street, NE, Washington, DC 20002-4242.

17. Ruan's book, *Sex in China* (1991), is an extremely valuable introduction to gay life in China.

18. In modern China, it is not only a term used in the Communist Party, but also by the Nationalist Party. In his last words the founding father of the modern republic, Sun Yusen, said: "The revolution has not succeeded, therefore our comrades need to continue to work hard."

19. *Tongzhi* has two characters, *tong* (the same) and *zhi* (will, interest, ideal, ambition, etc.). The Chinese word for homosexual(ity) has three characters, *tong* (the same), *xing* (sex, or gender) and *lian* (attach to, attracted to, and dating). *Tongzhi* starts with the same character as *tongxinglian*. It does not have a character denoting sex, which obviates associating gay people with their sexual behavior, but since the second character *zhi* has a broad range of meanings, sex and sexual attraction is not excluded. In some sense, *tongzhi* is similar to the English term "queer," a name that sexual minorities choose for themselves. However, there is a cultural difference. Chinese culture is very social and values collective interest over that of individuals. Intentionally associating oneself with a stigmatized notion like "queer" would be seen as being insincere and even anti-social. Therefore, the gay and lesbian community adopted one of the most sacred words in modern China to present themselves as equal members of the society.

20. One of them is *Their World: The Gay Male Population in China in Perspective*, by sociologist Li Yin He and her husband, writer Wang Xiao Bo, in 1992. In the book they reported the findings in their survey and interviews of 49 gay men in Beijing. The book was first published in Hong Kong because the authors could not find a publisher in Mainland China to accept their manuscript for such a sensitive topic (Samshasha, 1997), then by Shanxi Province People's Press. Part of the book's conclusions include things like "the majority of male-identified male homosexuals are people with narcissism" (p. 32), and "stable homosexual couples never lasts" (p. 70). Another book, the 700-page *Homosexuality*, is by Zhang Beichuan, a physician specializing in sexually transmitted disease. Although the author said that he did not approve of homosexuality, and a significant portion of the book is devoted to discussion of "treating homosexuality," it was one of the first books in China, after 1949, to look at the phenomenon and relative issues thoroughly in a relatively non-judgmental way. The author told me that some of the very homophobic remarks in the book were added by the publisher in order to publish the book.

21. The newsletter is devoted to AIDS education and communication between *tongzhi* and the general public; it is supported by the government and has a number of well-established scholars on its advisory board.

22. Since its debut in September 1997, to December 2001, it has published 113 issues plus 47 special additions, making it one of the most comprehensive on-line databanks for the Chinese *tongzhi* community. Its contents include a large quantity of translated materials from history to theories, as well as articles by Chinese authors on a broad range of topics related to homosexuality and *tongzhi* life. Given their politically low-key nature, gay men and lesbians in China feel safe and comfortable in pointing

out the articles and bringing them to gay bars to share with friends who do not have access to the Internet.

23. Some consider this the actual decriminalization of homosexuality (Lin, 2001). From that point on, police raiding of cruising sites and gay bars basically ceased, but in some areas, the neighborhood watchdogs still arrest and impose fines upon gay men found on those sites (Hunan TV, 2000).

24. It has been suggested that too much media coverage was partially responsible for the cancellation of the two events (Scat09, 2001; Wan, 2001).

25. In his research on the on-line tongzhi communication and AIDS prevention, Wan Yan Hai found more than 250 Chinese tongzhi web sites that were active and functional (Wan, e-mail communication, 2001).

26. He also visited with some of the CCMD task force members in different cities with an American gay activist and one of the founders of the national PFLAG, Lyle Henry. In addition, he convened two roundtable discussion sessions, inviting people in the gay and lesbian community to speak out. CCMD task force member Liu Hua Qing attended the sessions, and expressed his wish of researching gay and lesbians in the general population (Wan, 2001).

27. There I introduced him to American psychologist Douglas Kimmel, who had helped with the depathologization of homosexuality in Japan,. By then, there were already a handful Chinese *tongzhi* groups in the U.S. It was suggested to Wan that an umbrella organization be established to unite the community. Wan insisted that he did not want to be such an leader but he would want to do something for the community. In the e-mail discussion mainly among Wan, Lin Eryan and I, with some other people, Wan decided to settle in the research and educational area.

28. One of the most successful project of the CSSSM is the biweekly webzine *Tai Hong Man Tian Xia.*

29. *Homosexuality, a Side of the "Gender Personality*, by Li, Huichun (September 1, 1997), *Is Homosexuality Pathological?* by Cong, Zhong (October 1, 1997), *On the "Harmfulness" of Homosexuality–Deliberating with Mr. Jia, Yicheng*, by Lin, Eryan (December 31, 1997), and *Taking a Broader View in Studying the Phenomenon of Homosexuality and in Caring for the Homosexual Population*, by Zhang, Beichuan (February 1, 1997).

30. *Should Homosexuality Be Removed from the Chinese Diagnostic Criteria?* by Jia, Yicheng, (August 1997), *Keeping or Removing Homosexuality Should Depend on if It Is Pathological, Not the "National Condition,"* by Liang, Chuanshan, & Sun, Fengcai (September 1, 1997), *Removing Homosexuality Is Not Acceptable*, by Zhang, Zaifu (October 1, 1997), *We Should Not Delete the Diagnosis and Treatment of Homosexuality–Also Deliberating with Li Huichun*, by Long, Yi (November 1, 1997), and *Against "Turning on the Green Light" for Homosexuals*, by Jia, Yicheng (date unknown).

31. *We Need to Analyze "Homosexuality" in Particular*, by Lu Shengli, and *A Preliminary Exploration of the Psychology of Homosexuality*, by Hong, Xing (both November 1, 1997).

32. In fact, after the CCMD-III was changed in 2000, Jia spoke to the media to express his strong opposition.

33. To support his argument that there were too few homosexuals in China, he stated that even in labor reform camps specifically created for "homosexuals," the homosexual prisoners only composed about 1% of the total inmates. Arguably, this might be the first claim in China about the existence of labor reform camps designated to detain gay people.

34. The task force surveyed 51 subjects, using the Chinese version of the EPQ, MMPI, Diagnostic Scale for Mental Disorders (DSMD), the Social Function Rating Scales (SFRS), and their own questionnaire on mental health. The subjects included 34 men and 17 women, age range from 20 to 41; most had at least a high school education (some had a much higher level of schooling, but the report did not give specific percentages). The majority of them (44) never married; 4 were in heterosexual marriages, 3 had divorced.

35. When task force member Liu Huaqing visited the Lemon Tree Café to collect data, the gay and lesbian people there gave him mixed reactions (Wan, 2001). Some showed high respect and cooperated with the researcher, some were hostile but also filled out the questionnaires; some activists thought that the psychiatric label had nothing to do with who they were and disregarded the study.

36. This figure is higher than most other studies published in China. Most reports show that 30-40% gays and lesbians in China had suicidal ideation, and about 10% had suicide attempts. It is unclear if the difference is due to the wording of the questionnaires.

37. Given the mixed nature of the reported goals for therapy, it is unclear what facts the "effectiveness" data really conveyed. How much of the percentage was about self-acceptance, and how much was about change of sexual orientation?

REFERENCES

Chen, X. & Li, G. (1992), *Dangdai xinli weisheng [Contemporary Mental Health]*. Beijing: Chinese Social Science Press.

Chinese Psychiatric Association & the Neurological Hospital, Nanjing Medical University (1995), *Zhongguo jingshen jiping fanlei yu zhenduan biaozhun [The Chinese Classification of Mental Disorders (CCMD)]*. Nanjing, China: Southeast University Press.

Chou W. S. (1996), *Beijing Tongzhi Gushi [Stories of Tongzhis in Beijing]*. Hong Kong: Hong Kong Tongzhi Study Press.

Chou, W. S. (1997), *Post-Colonial Tongzhi*. Hong Kong: Hong Kong Tongzhi Press.

Cong, Z. & Gao, W. (1999), *Xinli yisheng jiezhen tongxinglian xianzhuang de chubu diaocha [A preliminary survey to the psychotherapists working with homosexual clients]*. *Chinese Journal of Behavioral Medical Science*, 3:225.

Cui, Z. (1997), *Taose zuichen [Pink Lips]*. Hong Kong: Worldson Books.

Ding, S. (1991), *Yang mou [The Open Plot]*. Hong Kong: The Nineties Monthly Press.

Fang, G. (1995), *Tongxinglian zai Zhongguo [Homosexual(ity) in China]*. Changchun, China: Jilin Province People's Press.

Gao, J., Pan, S., Yan, G. & Yang, X. (1985), *Zhongguo xinlixue shi [The History of Psychology in China]*. Beijing: The People's Educational Press.

Hunan TV (2000), *Let's Talk, 75.* (Transcript available at www.aizhi.org), December 20.

Lee, H. W. & Petzold, M. (1987), Psychology in the People's Republic of China. In: *Psychology Moving East: The Status of Western Psychology in Asia and Oceania,* eds. G. H. Blowers & A. M. Turtle. Boulder, CO: Westview Press, pp. 105-125.

Leinng (2001), *Shoujie tongxinglian dianyingjie jiang zai Beijing lakai weimu* [The first gay and lesbian movie festival will open its curtain in Beijing]. www.gaychinese. net, December, 20:29.

Li, H. (2001, March 28, 17:40), *Zhuanjia jieshi: tongxinglian bushi jingshenbingren* [Expert explains: homosexuals are not mental patients]. *Sanlian Shenghuo Zhoukan [Trinity Weekly].* On www.csssm.org/95gb.htm

Li, X., Xu, S. & Kuang, P. (1988), Thirty years of Chinese clinical psychology. *Int. J. Mental Health,* 16:3-21.

Li, Y. & Wang, X. (1992), *Tamen de shijie–zhongguo nan tongxinglian qunluo tongzhi* [*Their World: The Gay Male Population in China in Perspective*]. Taiyuan, China: Shanxi People's Press.

Lin, E. (2001), *Zhongguo tongxinglian feibinglihua yiweizhe shenmo* [What does depathologization of homosexuality in China mean?]. *Becoming Your Own Expert.* Beijing: AIZHI Action Project, and Taohong Man Tianxia Web Site <www.csssm.org>.

Liu, H., Zhang, P., Zou, Y., Liu, J., Li, X., Guo, F., Yao, F., Zhang, X. & Xu, H. (1999), *Tongxinglianzhe de xinli zhuangkuang jiqi xingcheng de yingxiang yinsu* (The psychological states of homosexuals and factors that influenced their formation). *Chinese Journal of Psychiatry, 32.*

Loo, J., ed. (1996), *Ta ta ta ta de gushi* [*His-His and Her-Her Stories*]. Hong Kong: Worldson Books.

Loo, J., ed. (1999), *Haren tongzhi xin duben* [*New Readings on Chinese Tongzhi*). Hong Kong: Worldson Books.

Lu, L., Pan, A., Chen, J., Liu, X., Lin, W. & Wang, H. (1992), Clinical analysis of 1000 homosexual cases. *Chinese Mental Health Journal,* 6:132-134.

Pan, S. (1993), China: Acceptability and effect of three kinds of sexual publication. *Arch. Sexual Behavior,* 22:59-71.

Qian, M. (1994), *Xinli zhiliao yu xinli zixun* [*Psychotherapy and Psychological Counseling*]. Beijing: Peking University Press.

Ruan, F. F. (1988), Male homosexuality in contemporary Mainland China. *Arch. Sexual Behavior,* 17:189-199.

Ruan, F. F. (1991), *Sex in China.* New York: Plenum Press.

Samshasha (1997), *Zhongguo tongxinglian shilu, zengding ben* [A History of Homosexuality in China, Expanded Edition]. Hong Kong: Rosa Winkel Press.

Scat09 (2001), *Shoujie quanguo tongzhi dianyingjie houhu huodong huo quxiao* [*The Later Activities of the First National Gay and Lesbian Movie Festival May Be Canceled*]. At <chinatongzhi@yahoogroups.com>.

Shen, Y. (1993), People's Republic of China. In: *International Handbook on Mental Health Policy,* ed. D. R. Kemp. Westport, CT: Greenwood, pp. 287-302.

Sleek, S. (1998), Chinese psychiatrists debate meaning of sex orientation. *APA Monitor,* September, p. 33.

Thornicroft, G. (1988), Contemporary psychiatry in China: Observations of a visiting professional. *Int. J. Mental Health,* 136:86-94.

Wan, Y. H. (1997), *Gay Rights and the Gay Movement in China in the 1990s*. Columbia University lecture, March 25.

Wan, Y. H. (2001), *Zhongguo tongxinglian zouxiang zhengchang* [Homosexuality becomes normal in China]. In: *Chengwei ziji de zhuanjia [Becoming One's Own Expert]*. Beijing: AIZHI Action Project & Taohong Man Tianxia Webzine (www.csssm.org).

Wu, C. & Chou, H., eds. (1996), *Women Huozhe* [We Are Alive]. Hong Kong: Hong Kong Tongzhi Study Press.

Xia, Z. & Zhang, M. (1988), History and present status of psychiatry in China. *Int. J. Mental Health*, 16:22-29.

Zhang, B. (1994), *Tong Xing Ai [Homosexuality]*. Jinan, China: Shandong Province Science and Technology Press.

Zhang, H. (1988), Psychological measurement in China. *Int. J. Psychol.*, 23:101-117.

Zhong, Y. (1991), *Zhongguo guonei xinli zhiliao yu zixun gaikuang* [A survey of psychotherapy and counseling in China]. *Chinese Mental Health Journal*, 5:38-40.

Homosexuality in India:
The Light at the End of the Tunnel

Suresh Parekh, MA

SUMMARY. This paper begins with a brief overview of sexuality and homosexuality in the Hindu civilization. In the sections that follow, the author discusses changing attitudes toward gay people, their legal status and the emergence of gay and lesbian organizations in modern India. As there is little psychiatric and psychological literature in India on the subject, the paper addresses the theoretical models used for understanding homosexuality in India on the basis of the few research studies published in psychiatry and psychology journals, unpublished reports, and interviews with psychiatrists and clinical psychologists. Finally, the paper concludes with some anecdotal accounts of gay people published in gay magazines or told by gay individuals regarding their experiences with mental health practitioners. *[Article copies available for a fee from The Haworth Document Delivery Service: 1-800-HAWORTH. E-mail address: <getinfo@haworthpressinc.com> Website: <http://www.HaworthPress.com> © 2003 by The Haworth Press, Inc. All rights reserved.]*

Suresh Parekh is Lecturer in Psychology, M.M.G. College, Junagadh, Gujarat, India.

The author wishes to express his sincere gratitude to: Dr. Ganpat Vankar, Professor and Head, Department of Psychiatry and Dr. B.K. Sinha, Assistant Professor of Clinical Psychology, B.J. Medical College, Ahmedabad; Dr. R. Brahmabhat, Consultant Sexologist, Mumbai; Dr. R. Kamat, Assistant Professor, Department of Psychiatry, K.E.M. Hospital, Mumbai; Dr. Dwarka Pershad and Dr. S.K. Verma, Retired Clinical Psychologists, PGIMER, Chandigarh; and Dr. Bholeshwar Mishra, Clinical Psychologist, Dayanand Medical College, Ludhiana. The author expresses his special gratitude to Mr. Sylvester Merchant and Mr. Manav, the trustees of 'Lakshya,' Rajpipla, and Mr. Ashok Row Kavi and Mr. Abhijit of 'Humsafar Trust,' Mumbai, for their extraordinary cooperation.

[Haworth co-indexing entry note]: "Homosexuality in India: The Light at the End of the Tunnel." Parekh. Suresh. Co-published simultaneously in *Journal of Gay & Lesbian Psychotherapy* (The Haworth Medical Press, an imprint of The Haworth Press, Inc.) Vol. 7, No. 1/2, 2003, pp. 145-163; and: *The Mental Health Professions and Homosexuality: International Perspectives* (ed: Vittorio Lingiardi, and Jack Drescher) The Haworth Medical Press, an imprint of The Haworth Press, Inc., 2003, pp. 145-163. Single or multiple copies of this article are available for a fee from The Haworth Document Delivery Service [1-800-HAWORTH, 9:00 a.m. - 5:00 p.m. (EST). E-mail address: getinfo@haworthpressinc.com].

http://www.haworthpressinc.com/store/product.asp?sku=J236
10.1300/J236v07n01_09

KEYWORDS. Antihomosexual attitudes, gay and lesbian organizazions, Hindu civilization, homosexuality, Indian Psychiatry, modern India, sexuality

SEXUALITY IN INDIA: A BRIEF OVERVIEW

Undoubtedly the Hindu civilization, among all other ancient civilizations, was the first to give sexuality, sexual activities and sexual pleasure a highly respectable place in all aspects of life, art, literature and even religion. Thousands of years ago, the seers and sages of ancient India suggested that there are four prime and principal aims or goals in the life of a person: (1) *Dharma* (duty of one's being), (2) *Artha* (acquisition of wealth), (3) *Kama* (pleasures of sex, sexual fulfillment), and (4) *Moksha* (release, liberation from the cycles of birth). A number of books called *Shastras* and *Sutras*, including *Kama Sutra*, were written by seers and sages in order to outline and teach the ways and means to achieve these four goals of human life.

For thousands of years, every Hindu and every Indian person has worshipped the natural *Lingam* stone installed in the *Yoni* (vagina) base as *Shiva*. *Lord Shiva*, who was considered the Great God, "the conqueror of death" and "the supreme yogi" in the ancient religious literature, is portrayed as *lingam*. The erect phallus, the *lingam* (penis) represents the great spirit in a state of excitement. "Shiva is pure existence, the immortal divine principle. Shiva is pure consciousness, unconditional and transcendental and Shiva is the deity of the mind, the lord of the yoga, master of the three worlds and the conqueror of death. The whole universe is created by the shakti of Shiva" (*Shiva Purana*, in Douglas and Slinger, 1979, p. 130). "The whole universe was created from the seed that poured from the erect *lingam* of Shiva during his love making. All the gods worship that *lingam*, the symbol of Lord Shiva, the supreme yogi" (*Mahabarata* in Douglas and Slinger, 1979, p. 34).

The Hindu have never considered sex apart from, or opposed to, spirituality or religion. They have never thought that love making was a sin, nor have they thought that love scenes were indecent, unworthy of being in temples and holy places. The sex act was given a place of honor and was intimately connected with all the arts. *Maithuna* (sexual congress/intercourse) was considered one of the main purposes of life, and religion encouraged the pursuit of this prime pleasure of life. Hence, erotic scenes formed an essential part of the scheme of decorative art. These scenes were the main theme or subject of the sculptors. All the sexual postures narrated in *Kama Sutra* and in other similar books, improved by the imagination of the sculptors, were depicted with extraordinary ability on the walls and pillars of world famous temples, including *Khajuraho*, *Konark* and *Modhera*.

The Hindu were probably the first among the ancients in studying sexual love as a natural emotion. The greatest ancient authority on the subject was *Vatsyayana*, a saint and a seer. His *Kama Sutra* (aphorisms of love) is thought even today to be a monumental work on the art and science of love not only by Indians, but also by Westerners. Every Hindu gentleman of the Middle Ages was expected to know something about the great masterpiece of love. The erotic sculptures of the great temples, the poems and dramas of great Indian writers show that they have a great knowledge of the art and science of love making. *Kama Sutra* enumerates sixty-four arts. The principal is the "art of love," without which no creative activity would be possible. "A person–says the *Kama Sutra* (Shastri, 1964, p. 53)–should study the sixty-four arts and sciences, as also the sixty-four aspects of sexual union."[1]

HOMOSEXUALITY IN INDIA

Religious as well as non-religious, written by saints or poets, the writings from the vedic and ancient period show that intense and passionate relationships or attachments between men and between women have always existed in India. Sometimes, and in some places, this kind of relationship was honored and praised as positive and even worthy of being imitated. In other periods and in other places, homosexuality was considered to be a very natural, normal and inevitable emotional aspect of human sexual life. For this reason, homosexual relationships were accepted and nobody paid much attention to them. For example, "homosexuality was not a condemned mode of sexual gratification when the temple sculptors of *Konark* and *Khajuraho* were depicting it in stone for all posterity to see" (Pradhan, Ayyar and Bagadia, 1982a, p. 182). Finally, there were other periods and places where homosexual love was punished and humiliated as unnatural, abnormal, unethical and immoral.

In their anthology, *Same-Sex Love in India*, Ruth Vanita and Saleem Kidwai (2000) have provided an extraordinary rich collection of writings on same-sex love from the ancient, medieval and modern Indian literature. They draw from epics like *Mahabharata, Ramayana, Panchatantra* and *Kathasaritsagara*; classics like *Kama Sutra, Arth Shastra, Manavdharmashastra* or *Manu Smriti*; Puranic literature like *Bhagvata Purana, Skanda Purana, Shiva Purana*, and Ayurvedic or Indian medical texts like *Charaka Samhita, Sushruta Samhita* and many more. Douglas and Slinger (1979) write:

> In ancient India, it was considered normal for woman to have intimate relationships with other women. Close physical contact between women has always been considered normal and healthy in Eastern Cultures. Sisters or women friends would commonly share the same bed. The word *sakhi* or 'girl friend' is related to *Shakti*, the vital female power principle,

the raw Energy of Tantra. To have a *Sakhi* as a companion was considered vitalizing, auspicious and social. It was widely believed that such sisterhoods strengthened the femininity of all participants. A *sakhi* added her own qualities and experiences to those of her 'sister.' Often a woman and her *sakhi* were inseparable. Sapphic activities within such sisterhoods were considered normal and are frequently portrayed in Indian art . . . The *Ramayana*, an important Hindu epic, contains an account of a menage in which sapphic sex is poetically described: There were innumerable women lying on rugs, who had fallen asleep after spending the night in sensual play. Their breath was subtly perfumed with sweetened wine. Some of the girls savored each other's lips as they dreamed, as if they were their masters. Their aroused passions drove these lovely sleeping women to make love to their companions. Some slept in their rich garments, propped up on bracelet laden arms; some lay across their companions, on their bellies, their breasts, their thighs, their backs, clinging amorously to one another with arms entwined, the slender wasted women lay together in sweet intoxicated sleep . . . The *Kama Sutra* describes how women can use their mouths on each other's *Yonis* (vaginas) and describes also many ways of satisfying sexual desires with bulbs, roots or fruits which have the same shape as the lingam. (in Douglas and Slinger, 1979, pp. 326-327)

In different periods and in different vernacular languages of India, a number of terms were used for homosexual behaviors and for those who engaged in those behaviors. Terms like "heterosexual," "homosexual" and "bisexual" were imported into India from the west in the late nineteenth and in the early twentieth century. Prior to that, in some Indian texts, more then two gender classes were categorized. In *Kama Sutra*, Vatsyayana attempted to categorize the types of sexual behaviors and the people who express these behaviors. *Tritiya Prakriti* (literally "third nature") is *napunsaka*, neither man nor woman. These individuals obtain pleasure from oral sex with men. *Purushayita* is a "woman acting like a man." The term *Auparashtika* is used for oral sex. *Charaka Samhita* states, "The male who gets an erection and is able to have intercourse with a woman only after having had his anus penetrated by another male is *Gudyoni napunsak*."[2]

There is debate among scholars whether the practice of anal sex was indigenous to India or arrived with the Muslims. "Anal sex between men was unheard of in India until the Muslim invasions" (Douglas and Slinger, 1979, p. 338). "Given the widespread popular assumption in modern India that boy prostitution, eunuchs and even anal sex appeared only following the advent of Islam, it is important to note that in pre-Islamic texts, men and boy prostitutes and dancers who service men are represented in descriptive, non-condemning terms, as normally present in court and in daily life and as evidence of the affluence and splendor of urban culture" (Vanita and Kidwai, 2000, p. 27). "Given the popular misconception that penetrative anal sex was introduced in India after Muslim rule, it is important to note that it is mentioned in the *Kama Sutra* as one of the many types of copulation: 'copulation below, in the anus, is practiced by southern people' (our translation)" (Vanita and Kidwai, 2000, p. 48). "The institution of male prostitution is said to owe its origin to the Muslim rulers of olden days who used to keep 'boys' for sodomy. They also brought this evil to India, and in old Muslim capital towns of India, boy prostitutes used to sit in open windows like female prostitutes, soliciting customers. In pre-independence days, such a scene was pretty common in cities like Lucknow or Delhi" (Varma, 1979, p. 97).

What is known, however, is that during the period of Muslim rule (precisely, from the beginning of the eighteenth century to the end of the first half of the nineteenth century), the profession of male prostitution was at its peak. Mishra (1974) notes, "In India, unnatural same sex intercourses were started by Muslims and were practiced before and during the Mugal period. In the eighteenth century, it had become a fashion in the absence of any ethical, religious or administrative control" (p. 67). He goes on to say the "Ethical breakdown of society [sic] was not limited to Delhi only, and Faizabad and Lucknow were bigger and very active centers. The poet Mir Hasan Dehalvi has given a scholarly description which he himself has witnessed: 'Somewhere standing are *launde* (boys) with make up, around them have arrived the *laundebaz* (boy lovers)' " (p. 68).

The capacity of seducing a boy was considered an art of the *ishkbaz* (boy lover) and was also a praiseworthy topic of discussion among friends. In order to attain this goal, the "hunter of boys" implemented various tricks. For example, in order to entrap a handsome and smart boy, Nazeer Akbarbadi, in his poem *Bayan* (Urdu word for a weaver bird), described in detail how he brought a beautiful *bayan* and doing so he made the boy very jealous. "Then, in order to show a more miraculous thing, 'a tree of seashell,' he brought the boy to an isolated place and succeeded in the evil act."[3]

As we move to contemporary times, there have been no attempts to undertake large scale surveys of patterns of sexual behavior among Indian men or women, such as the American studies conducted by Kinsey (Kinsey, Pomeroy and Martin, 1948; Kinsey et al., 1953) and Hite (1977, 1981). Hence it is impossible to reliably estimate the actual numbers or percentage of homosexual people (both gay and lesbian) in the Indian population. Chan et al. (1998) estimates that "Men having Sex with Men" (MSM) range between 12.5 million and 37.4 million. This figure is based upon Kinsey's statistics of the frequency of homosexuality in men who fall between 3 and 6 on the Kinsey Scale which were applied to the provisional Indian census figures of 1991. However, even if only 2% of the Indian population is exclusively homosexual, then the actual number might reach beyond 20 million as the population of India surpassed one billion in the 21st century.

ANTIHOMOSEXUAL ATTITUDES IN INDIA

Insofar as homosexuality has never been totally accepted in India, anti-homosexual attitudes in various forms and to various degrees have existed and been expressed throughout the history of India. The forms of antihomosexual attitudes ranged from ignorance to insults to physical attacks and to punishment. According to one report, "at most times and places in pre-nineteenth-century India, love between women and between men, even when disapproved of, was not actively persecuted. As far as we know, no one has ever been executed for homosexuality in India" (Vanita and Kidwai, 2000, p. xviii). Nevertheless, the range and severity of antihomosexual responses has differed in different periods and places, depending upon an individual's age, caste and genders. Some examples:

> In the *Arthashastra*, there is a wide category of *ayoni*, or non-vaginal sex (as it is named in other texts such as the *Mahabharata*) which, whether with a man or a woman, is punishable with the first fine. The first fine is the lowest fine payable in grades for robberies of three types and of not very high value . . . The *Manusmriti* appears even less judgmental in its famous prescription that a man who has sex with a man, or with a woman in a cart pulled by a cow, in water or by day, should bathe with his clothes on (XI:175). XI:174 prescribes that a man who sheds his semen in non-human females, in a man, in a menstruating woman, in something other than a vagina or in water has to perform a minor penance consisting of eating the five products of the cow and keeping a one night fast. This is the same penance prescribed for stealing articles of little value. (Vanita and Kidwai, 2000, p. 25)

> India's Hindu culture, which is a shame culture rather than a guilt culture, treats homosexual practice with secrecy but not with malice . . . The passive gay is subjected to the same humiliation while walking down a street as a woman is in India . . . This hatred of homosexual people, I think, goes back to the Judaic, Zoroastrian, Christian, Islamic injunctions against oral or anal sex as being 'unproductive,' 'sterile.' (Merchant, 1999, pp. xii-xv)

Until recent times, "The rights of gay people is a subject little mentioned, rarely discussed in this country. In fact, until the marriage of Leela and Urmila, two women constables from the Madhya Pradesh police was announced, the subject of homosexuality was hardly mentioned in the media, much less has it come up for decision before our courts" (Jaising, 1988, p. 24). Leela and Urmila were discharged from the Madhya Pradesh police force for what was termed "unauthorized absence from duty." However, it may be that the real reason for their removal from service is the fact that they were lesbians and had announced that they would marry each other. Shamona Khanna (1992) reports that police entrapment–and worse–of gays is common: "Every evening, plain-clothes policemen spread out over gay meeting places in all metropolitan cities to entrap, humiliate, extort money from and even force sex on gay men under the threat of criminal prosecution" (p. 6).

Much of what is known about antihomosexual attitudes in India is anecdotal. The following was published in the *Bombay Dost*, a gay magazine of the Humsafar Trust of Mumbai:

> Four years back when I was new to the scene, I had a miserable experience while cruising at a railway station in town. Someone I fancied responded positively and I dutifully followed him to the dark and desolate streets leading to Marine Drive. We started talking and I failed to notice that he was actually answering in monosyllables. A little later, when no one was around, this man announced: 'Your game is over and I am a policeman. You people have infested this station and we are cleaning it up these days.' I was totally taken by surprise. He relentlessly gripped my hand and kept dragging me to a police van that was supposedly parked nearby. In my panic, I forgot that I had actually not done anything wrong so far. I kept rattling 'sorry' in Hindi, English and Marathi to win over his leniency for at least 'this time.' He mercilessly refused to listen to me and I was totally terrorized thinking about the impending police van. Finally he agreed to leave me 'this time' for a sum of two thousand five hundred rupees, which further agitated me. I showed him my wallet to support my contention and he took out my company ID-card. He said that I could manage the balance of money after leaving my watch and the ID-card as security. My optimism rose slightly and I requested that he take all the money in my wallet and that he give me twenty rupees to get back home. He took four hundred rupees and gave me five rupees back saying, 'Forget taxi fare. I'd better not see you roaming in this area again.' (Nishant, 1999, p. 11)

CHANGING SCENARIO

Today, in India, there are many organizations promoting the civil rights of gay men and lesbians.[4] ABVA (*AIDS Bhedbhav Virodhi Andolan* [AIDS

Antidiscrimination Movement]), for example, is a Delhi based non-governmental organization, working for the welfare of AIDS victims, AIDS awareness, gay rights, etc., submitted a charter of 16 demands to the Petition Committee of Parliament to improve the status of homosexuality in India. Some of the demands included: decriminalization of sodomy by repealing section 377 of the Indian Penal Code (IPC), legalization of same sex-marriages, setting up a commission for documenting human rights violations against homosexuality, reformation of police policy for ending institutionalized harassment of gay people, etc.

ABVA filed a petition in the Delhi High Court in April 1994 to challenge the legality of section 377 of the Indian Penal Code (IPC) because it violates article 226 of the Indian Constitution. Apart from section 377, there is no other law in the IPC which deals with homosexuality or homosexual behaviors between men or women. IPC section 377, which was originally enacted by the British in 1860, reads as follows: "Unnatural offences: whoever voluntarily has carnal intercourse against the order of nature with any man, woman or animal, shall be punished with imprisonment for a term which may extend to ten years and shall be liable to fine." Section 377 does not call homosexuality per se illegal, but sodomy–either homosexual or heterosexual–is punishable. Since its inception, the sodomy law has rarely been used, but as in many other countries, its presence hangs like a sword of Damocles over gay and lesbian people in India.

The last decade of the twentieth century has witnessed the establishment of a number of gay and/or lesbian organizations. Some of them are openly registered and recognized by the government and they are comprised of self-identified gay and lesbian people in many parts of the country. One is *Humsafar Trust* of Mumbai in Maharashtra state, and the other is *Lakshya Trust* of Rajpipla in Gujarat state.

Humsafar Trust was established in early 1990 and was registered in 1994. The trust has made great efforts to raise awareness on male sexual health. The work of the trust has four main components: community work, outreach to gay and MSM groups, advocacy on gender and sexuality issues concerning sexual minorities, and research into sexuality and gender issues. The trust successfully organized the first South Asian Gay conference in 1994. In 1995, the trust became a member of the International Gay and Lesbian Human Rights Commission (IGLHRC) and of the International Lesbian and Gay Association (ILGA). *Lakshya Trust* was established in 2000. In the same year, the trust organized the first gay conference in Gujarat. In this three day conference, gay people from at least 11 districts of Gujarat participated. The trust is successfully undertaking projects on self empowerment, STD and HIV/AIDS awareness, etc. with grants from various government agencies. Since their inception, both of the above trusts have managed to coordinate themselves with the government, the public health authorities, medical institutions and other social groups for different projects. More importantly, however, both trusts have provided emotional and psychological support for many gay people who want to come out from their closeted lives.

UNDERSTANDING HOMOSEXUALITY: PREVAILING THEORETICAL MODELS[5]

Indian academicians in the field of psychiatry and psychology have preserved an almost complete silence on the subject of homosexuality, notwithstanding that the subject has a history of at least three thousand years in this land. Indian behavioral scientists, psychiatrists and psychologists have avoided writing on homosexuality and thus there is not a single book on the subject that has been written by them.

What may be the first book on the subject was published in 1977 by the legendary Indian mathematics wizard Shakuntala Devi (1977).[6] Vanita and Kidwai (2000) have given a fair account of the contents of the book. The book reviewed homosexuality in history, in relation to law, psychiatry, different religions and cultures, with a detailed account of surveys carried out by Western scientists. "The book ends with a call for decriminalization as well as 'full and complete acceptance, not tolerance and not sympathy' by the heterosexual population, which will enable homosexuals to come out of hiding and lead dignified, secure lives" (Vanita and Kidwai, 2000, p. 205).

Another publication is by ABVA, although in booklet form, and is entitled *Less Than Gay* (1991). It contains interviews with gay people, surveys, the legal, social, medical, and cultural context of homosexuality, and also attempts to address myths about homosexuality.

The *Indian Journal of Clinical Psychology* is an official publication of the Indian Association of Clinical Psychologists. The journal started in 1974 and is regularly published every six months. Volume 28, No. 1 (March, 2001) is a special issue containing abstracts of all research papers published between 1974 and 2000. Out of 829 research papers published in 27 volumes of this journal, only two papers were about homosexuality: Rangaswamy[7] (1982) and Nammalvar, Rao and Ramasubramaniam (1983). There was also one editorial on *Psychological Sequelae of AIDS* (Gupta, 1989) in which homosexuality is not the main subject, but is specifically mentioned.

In "Modification of Homosexual Behaviour: A Case Report," Nammalvar, Rao and Ramasubramaniam (1983) do not clearly describe the patient, but the details of the patient's history given as background suggest that they believe he learned his homosexual orientation and preference during adolescence, when he was conditioned by anal intercourse. They go on to say:

[The patient] was indulging in homosexual behavior from age 14, when he was placed in a boarding school for the first time. On the first occasion he was made to observe his friends having homosexual intercourse and grew up curious about it. He initiated the homosexual act as an active partner with a junior member of the school. Later he was indulging in such behavior periodically. He started choosing classmates who were around the age of 14. He continued to be an active partner and had never opted for a passive role. Even after leaving school, he used to pick up boys from his village. As a landlord he could command boys in the neighborhood. Later, at the age of 22, when his mother started seeking [a marriage] alliance for him, he became alarmed. For the first time he wanted to try heterosexual acts. But he could not succeed. There was no penile erection, but at the same time he succeeded in anal intercourse with the same girl [sic] . . . Significant improvement was noticed in the reduction of homosexual fantasies and behavior in just 20 sessions of treatment. (pp. 35-38)

In a review of all the articles in the *Indian Journal of Psychiatry* between 1982 and 1995, there were only four research papers on homosexuality: Pradhan, Ayyar and Bagadia (1982a,b), Mehta and Nimgaonkar (1983), and Jiloha (1984). Here too, there is only one editorial addressing AIDS that makes any specific mention of homosexuality (Agarwal, 1990).

Pradhan, Ayyar and Bagadia (1982a) present the details and the treatment outcomes of thirteen treatments with homosexual patients (diagnosed according to ICD-8 criteria). They used behavior modification techniques, but they neither present the history of these patients nor do they discuss the presumed causes of the subjects' homosexuality. The authors state that "eight (61%) of our thirteen patients showed very good improvement and out of these, four got married or engaged after treatment and had successful sexual intercourse with a female on a six month to one year follow up" (p. 81). In their second paper (Pradhan, Ayyar and Bagadia, 1982b), they again present a psychiatric study of thirteen homosexual patients. They report that the patients show no clinical evidence of hormone deficiency. They also theorize that early childhood experiences were important in the causation of homosexuality: an early channeling of the sexual drive to same sex objects due to homosexual seduction and subsequent practice was felt to play an important role.

Mehta and Nimgaonkar (1983) present the report of the treatment of six homosexual patients (five males and one female). There is no discussion of the history and the presumed causes of the homosexual behavior in these people. They claimed to have achieved successful "reorientation" in four subjects.

Jiloha (1984) presents the case history of a patient that concludes with a psychodynamic explanation of the patient's homosexuality:

Mr. S.T. has a narcissistic personality. He experiences an intense and confusing oedipal situation which is still unresolved and active. There is evidence of castration anxiety, guilt which manifests in the form of searching for a partner of the same sex. The patient felt seduced by his mother and felt threatened after the arrival of his younger sister which resulted in hatred for young females. The other possible reason for his homosexuality could be his unconscious desire to prove himself more powerful and masculine than other males (which represent the father figure). (p. 404)

Agarwal (1990), in his editorial on "Strategies for primary prevention of AIDS," writes:

Often homosexuality is considered to be some kind of wickedness and therefore frowned upon. In our country homosexuality is considered to be an offense. However, some behaviorists view homosexuality as an innate variation for which the sufferer himself is not responsible. It is a quirk of fate that a small minority develop homosexual orientation. As the society does not allow them to satisfy their needs of intimacy they have to fulfill their emotional needs in a clandestine manner due to the fact that stable relationships cannot be formed while frequent casual contacts increase the risk of infection. Instead of branding them as criminals or offenders, society should accept their deviation as part of normal spectrum of behavior so that they may fulfill their emotional needs in a legitimate manner and as such may not be driven to casual sex. (pp. 209-210)

Other than the articles mentioned above, a review of the *Indian Journal of Psychological Medicine* (issues published between 1986 to 1995), the *Journal of Community Guidance and Research*, and the *Journal of Personality and Clinical Studies* revealed no other research papers dealing with homosexuality.[8]

There are, however, discussions of homosexuality taking place in popular magazines and newspapers. Recently, an article by Jahnavi Contractor entitled, *Your Horoscope Can Determine if You Are Homosexual,* was published in *The Sunday Times of India.* The article was based on an interview with a well-known Indian sexologist, Dr. Prakash Kothari. According to Dr. Kothari, India's eminent astronomer and astrologer Varahmihir (6th century A.D.) mentions homosexuality as a trait observed in individuals whose horoscope indicates a particular planetary condition (when Venus and Saturn face each other). As reported in the article, Dr. Kothari carried out a study at King Edward Memorial Hospital and Department of Sexual Medicine, at the Medical College of Mumbai. Eighty homosexual patients' horoscopes were charted out by an expert astrologer and in a majority of cases, barring a few exceptions that Varahmihir has mentioned, most had the peculiar planetary position that he has described. Dr. Kothari concludes that if modern studies have pointed out that homosexuality is a genetic trait and is congenital, astrology also seems to indicate that homosexuality is inborn!

What follows are excerpts from some of my interviews with mental health professionals. The interviews were semi-structured and focused mainly on understanding the professional's attitudes towards homosexuality and the specific theoretical model followed. During the interviews, I attempted to find out not only the personal attitude towards homosexuality, but also the attitude of the professional fraternity of that particular region.

> Homosexuality is not an abnormality but it is a way of life. In a conservative country like India, persons with homosexual orientation face very strong social stigma and are marginalized . . . We personally feel that homosexuals should be treated with dignity and honor like any other persons in our society. They should be allowed to be part of the mainstream of social living rather than marginalized . . . We accept a bio-psycho-social approach to understanding homosexuality, but we would prefer an eclectic approach to addressing this issue. (Dr. G. K. Vankar, Professor and Head, and Dr. B. K. Sinha, Assistant Professor of Clinical Psychology, Department of Psychiatry, B. J. Medical college, Ahmedabad)

> [Homosexuality] is a normal variant of sexuality. Homosexuals are a minority but they are normal. There is also the fact that after knowing the scientific facts about homosexuality, many doctors and psychiatrists still feel this as an abnormality and they are not comfortable with it at a personal as well as professional level . . . There isn't any perfect theoretical model. There is no model which is sufficient to explain every homosexual person or which can be applied to every homosexual. (Dr. Raj Brahmbhatt, Consulting Sexologist, Consultant in charge, Sexuality Education Counseling Research Therapy/Training (SECRT) Mumbai, associated with the Family Planning Association of India)

> Homosexuality is not an abnormality. I feel that most of the psychiatrists of this region believe that it is not an abnormality. It is more behavioral rather than biological. Causes of homosexuality vary from one person to another, and from a specific situation to another situation. Children who are staying in hostels are more susceptible to homosexual encounters and for adolescents it is one of the outlets of sexuality. (Dr. Ravindra Kamat, Asst. Professor of Psychiatry, K.E.M. Hospital, Mumbai)

It is not a mental disorder or abnormality. It is a matter of habit and preference. The genesis of this habit can be described on the basis of learning during childhood or in the past as a whole . . . No single theoretical model can be used as an explanation for every homosexual individual. Probably the latest theory of learning can explain the sexual preference of an individual. The psychoanalytic model and biological model are also useful but they cannot be fully used because of their poor validity and lack of more authenticated research. (Dr. Dwarka Pershad and Dr. S. K. Verma, retired Professors of Clinical Psychology, Post-Graduate Institute of Medical Education and Research (PGIMER), Chandigarh)

Homosexuality is an abnormality if and when it is stressful and interferes with the day to day activities of an individual. But if it is not interfering with the individual's progress, with his or her adjustment and when it is not stressful, then it is normal. I think most of the clinical psychologists have the same opinion or attitude towards homosexuality . . . I do accept various theoretical models to explain homosexuality. Psychological models are sufficient to explain certain categories of homosexuals. Biological models do have some explanation for homosexuality. (Dr. Bholeshwar Mishra, Clinical Psychologist, Dayanand Medical College, Ludhiana, Punjab)

TELLING TALES:
SEEING A MENTAL HEALTH PROFESSIONAL

This section includes some anecdotal accounts of attitudes toward gay people expressed by mental health and other professionals.[9] They are presented as illustrative of some of the difficulties gay and lesbian patients face when seeking treatment. The following experience of a medical resident was published in *Bombay Dost*[10] (Samuel, 1990):

It was my turn to present the usual weekly departmental seminar and I had chosen the topic, 'Disease in the Male Homosexual.' I wanted to speak on the above topic. Mainly because (1) it was interesting and topical, (2) because clinicians were not prepared to diagnose sexually transmitted diseases in gays in light of their sexual preferences and (3) clinicians are not prepared to accept gay patients, at least without feeling a slight degree of hostility or even revulsion. I, with the help of Sanjay Siddharth, Psychiatrist, KEM and ARK, collected enough material on the psychosocial, cross cultural and medical aspects of gay behavior. The lecture outlined the fact that homosexuality has existed from time immemorial. We had come prepared to face a certain amount of hostility from the lecturers and seminar readers. Within two minutes, a seminar lecturer objected stating he had not come to listen to the APA (American Psychiatric Association) clarification on homosexuality and the universality of gay behavior. I replied that a recent survey in America showed that 60 per cent of doctors were uncomfortable treating homosexual patients and that I was only trying to lessen the hostility and desensitize them to the subject. I had also replied that microbiology is not just taking throat swabs for gonorrhea but something more. Within five minutes, people started walking out and I was urged by the seminar reader to hasten my lecture. I just folded all my papers and transparencies and switched off the projector.

Anil was 21 year old. He decided to see a psychiatrist after finding he was sexually attracted to men. The psychiatrist gave him an appointment. For the first session of over an hour, the psychiatrist charged Rs. 1050 [US$ 22] as a consultancy fee. The psychiatrist called him again the following week for the treatment. The treatment consisted of aversion therapy where he was shown pictures of nude men and given mild shock. He was then shown pictures of nude women and given his favorite sweets. This treatment was given for six sessions and charged Rs. 5000 [US$ 104]. He was not cured; instead he had a nervous breakdown.[11]

'Yes Ma! . . . I think I am gay,' I said without batting an eyelash. I was astonished for having uttered that, and with such apparent ease too. It was as if those feelings of fear, apprehension and self-loathing that had been bottled up inside me for as long as I could remember, that had, like a fragile dam of mud vainly trying to hold back the relentless force of a mighty river, suddenly burst apart. Since I was my Mother's only unmarried child she had been trying to get me married for the last year. She even took me to a psychiatrist, who, on hearing me out, threw up his hands and said, 'There is nothing you or I can do to change your son. The only thing you can do is to accept him as he is.' Mummy was not the sort who would give in easily. 'Who the hell is this quack anyway? He thinks he knows you better than me. Mothers are the best psychiatrists and I know as your mother that you can be changed. I shall not rest till I change you,' she declared. (Yogi, 1996)

I decided to burst the bubble after 15 years in which I had isolated myself from the rest of the world. I decided to step out of the wrapped view of the world that I was seeing into the real world, where I could breathe freely. I asked my doctor and he told me that it is best for you to come out. I clarified my queries about being converted to the main stream heterosexual life style. I had heard this was being performed by some practitioners, but I was told that they do more harm than good to your peace of mind and general well being. I dropped the idea. I felt comfort in the fact that it has been proved that being gay is not a disease and it is as natural as being heterosexual. (Rajat, 1999)

Rahul, a 28 year old man, comes from a typical middle class Gujarati family. He is more attached to his mother than his father. His gay life is active but closeted. The pressure to marry from family members and even society is relentless. His father is an educated and kind man. So, he comes out to his father. He tries to convince his father that he wishes to be as he is. Though his father is disturbed, he tries to make Rahul believe that this is merely a passing phase of life and that, in due course, everything will be all right. His father brings him to a psychiatrist. Rahul tells the psychiatrist about his homosexuality. The psychiatrist has a positive and affirmative attitude towards homosexuality and thus he talks to Rahul's father and tries to convince him that his son's sexual orientation is natural and that he should accept it and adjust to his son's lifestyle. His father accepts the reality and Rahul is happy.[12]

Not all psychiatrists are as accepting as Rahul's. In a commemorative publication of the Indian Psychiatric Society North Zone, R. M. Varma, writes:

Not infrequently non-normative alliances, while having the potential to provide an 'illusive' emotional fulfillment, result in dehumanization of human relations, besides other more drastic consequences. The evidence of such phenomena can be seen in homosexuality, lesbianism, sado-masochism and sex-related crimes like gang rape, incest and pedophilia. (Varma, 2000, pp. 28-29)

In 2001 the *Indian Express* published an article entitled "Indian Shrinks Treat Homosexuality as a Disease." The article noted that:

The first complaint in the country of a human rights violation against homosexuals has been filed with the National Human Rights Commission [NHRC]. Shaleen Rakesh, a gay activist of the Naz Foundation India Trust, a HIV/AIDS and sexual health awareness agency, has filed the complaint on the ground that the Indian Psychiatric Society has not formally recognized homosexuality as normal behavior. The complaint says gays who consult a psychiatrist are often told that homosexuality is a mental disease and needs to be cured. Rakesh says, 'There have been instances when psychiatrists have put gay men through unimaginable physical and psychological torture to try and convert them to heterosexuality by using techniques such as hypnosis, aversion therapy and, in some cases, even shock treatment. This is often done purely with the aim of making money . . . Gay men consult doctors because of the extreme emotional and psychological turmoil caused by Indian society's homophobia and not because homosexuality is a pathological or clinical disorder. This is something that psychiatrists have to recognize'. Dr. Sandeep Vohra, president of the Delhi Psychiatric Society, says psychiatrists all over the country recognize that homosexuality is not a mental illness: 'When gay men come to us with their problems, we tell them to accept their sexuality. We do not treat it as a mental disorder. If these gay men have had encounters with doctors forcing aversion therapy, it's because they are going to the wrong people; general physicians and psychologists who do not know how to handle the situation. It is true, however that some old timers in the psychiatric society may not have accepted homosexuality.' (*Indian Express*, 2001)

In response to the complaint, the NHRC wrote to Rakesh that the Commission did not find it necessary to take any further action in the matter and had closed the file. "Dr. Sandeep Vohra, Senior Consulting Psychiatrist of the Apollo Hospital and President of the Delhi Psychiatric Society as well as a member of the Indian Psychiatric Society has this to say: 'I cannot comment on the position of the NHRC but our stand remains the same. Homosexuality is not a disease, and we will continue to treat it that way" (*The Pioneer*, 2001).

GAY AND LESBIAN MENTAL HEALTH PROFESSIONALS

How many Indian mental health practitioners are openly gay? I enquired of every psychiatrist and clinical psychologist working in the places I visited while writing this paper. For the time being, I have been unable to find any openly gay or lesbian mental health professionals in India.

Perhaps, not too far in the future, we will see a light at the end of the tunnel.

NOTES

1. Later, a number of literary works were written by well-known pundits including Koka's *Rati Rahasya* [*Mysteries of Passion*] (Comfort, 1965; Upadhyaya, 1965), and Kalyanmalla's *Anang Rang* [*Theater of the Love God*] (Arbuthnot and Burton, 1964; Burton, 1963; Ray, 1944). Well known poets and playwrights like Kalidasa, Bhartruhari and Jagannath also have written literary masterpieces on the art of love (Patel, 1984; Savaliya, 2002).

2. Personal communication from V. N. Bhatt on the English translation of the Sanskrit text from the *Charak Samhita*, Gujarat Ayurvedic College, Junagadh.

3. Personal communication from K. P. Baku on the English translation of the Hindi text *Uttar Bharatmen Muslim Samaj* (see Mishra, 1974).

4. Among the more prominent organizations are Humsafar Trust, *Bombay Dost* magazine, and Stree Sangam (lesbian) in Bombay; Humrahi (gay men's group and help line), Sangini (lesbian group and help line), ABVA (AIDS Bhedbhav Virodhi Andolan, or AIDS Antidiscrimination Movement), and NAZ Foundation India Trust (both anti-AIDS) in Delhi; Good As You in Bangalore; Counsel Club in Calcutta; Friends India in Lucknow. See the ABVA Report (1991) and the updated resource guide, *Humjinsi*, edited by Bina Fernandez (1999).

5. In order to collect relevant resources to address this issue, I concentrated my efforts mainly on considering the following three sources: (1) Books and scientific journals published in India in the fields of psychology and psychiatry, and unpublished studies on gay and lesbian life; (2) Non-academic (popular) published literature; and (3) Personal interviews with psychiatrists and clinical psychologists.

6. In three university libraries where I sought out the book, it was not in the index; in another library it was in the index, but it was not issued to any reader nor was it in its designated place. I also contacted the publisher was informed that the book was out of print and unavailable.

7. Rangaswamy's (1982) paper was not available for study at the time of preparation of this paper. Its title, "Difficulties in Arousing and Increasing Heterosexual Responsiveness in a Homosexual," alludes to the "reparative therapy" nature of the author's research interest.

8. I have made serious attempts to find out whether any doctoral and post-doctoral research work has been carried out in psychology and psychiatry departments of universities and medical institutions of different regions of India. These attempts were made through long distance telephone calls to the friends and even friends' friends who work in the fields of psychology and psychiatry as well as through personal visits to the places mentioned in the acknowledgment. Everyone has responded, "I have no knowledge of any doctoral work on homosexuality in my university/institution/region."

9. Some of them have been first published in the magazine *Bombay Dost* while others have been narrated by Mr. Sylvester Merchant of *Lakshya Trust* and by Mr. Ashok Row Kavi of *Humsafar Trust*. The individuals interviewed by the author have given their permission to quote them.

10. The report is by M. Samuel, Resident in Microbiology, Seth G. S. Medical college in the first quarter of 1990. This is his report of a seminar held at the Department of Microbiology, KEM Hospital.

11. This story was told by Mr. Ashok Row Kavi.

12. This story was told by Mr. Sylvester Merchant of *Lakshya Trust*.

REFERENCES

ABVA (AIDS Bhedbhav Virodhi Andolan), (1991), *Less than Gay*. Report ABVA.

Arbuthnot, F. F.. & Burton, R., eds. & trans. (1964), *Ananga Ranga: The Hindu Art of Love by Kalyana Malla*. New York: Medical Press.

Agarwal, A. K. (1990), Editorial: Strategies for primary prevention of AIDS. *Indian J. Psychiatry*, 32(3):209-210.

Burton, R., trans. (1963), *Hindu Art of Love (Ananga Ranga)*. London: Neville Spearman.

Chan, R., Row Kavi, A., Carl, G., Khan, S., Oetomo, D., Tan, M. L. & Brown, T. (1998), HIV and men who have sex with men: Perspectives from selected Asian countries. *AIDS*, 12 (Supp/B):559-568.

Comfort, A., ed. & trans. (1965), *The Koka Shastra: Medieval Indian Writings on Love (Ratirahsya of Kokkoka)*. New York: Stein & Day.

Contractor, J. (2002), Your horoscope can determine if you are homosexual. *The Sunday Times of India*, January, 20:3.

Douglas, N. & Slinger, P. (1979), *Sexual Secrets: The Alchemy of Ecstasy*. New York: Destiny Books.

Fernandez, B., ed. (1999), *Humjinsi*. Mumbai: India Center for Human Rights.

Gupta, S. C. (1989), Editorial: Psychological sequelae of AIDS. *Indian J. Clinical Psychology*, 16(1):v-vi.

Hite, S. (1977), *The Hite Report*. New York: Dell.

Hite, S. (1981), *The Hite Report on Male Sexuality*. New York: Alfred A. Knopf.

Indian Express (2001), Indian shrinks treat homosexuality as a disease, June 20. Reprinted in *Pukaar*, 35, October 2001, p. 8.

Jaising, I. (1988), Gay rights. *The Lawyers*, Feb-Mar, pp. 24-25.

Jiloha, R. C. (1984), A case of unusual sexual perversion. *Indian J. Psychiatry*, 26(4):403-404.

Khanna, S. (1992), Gay rights. *The Lawyers*, June, pp. 4-9.

Kinsey, A., Pomeroy, W. & Martin, C. (1948), *Sexual Behavior in the Human Male*. Philadelphia, PA: Saunders.

Kinsey, A., Pomeroy, W., Martin, C. & Gebhard, P. (1953), *Sexual Behavior in the Human Female*. Philadelphia, PA: Saunders.

Mehta, M. & Nimgaonkar, S. (1983), Homosexuality: A study of treatment and outcome. *Indian J. Psychiatry*, 25(3):235-238.

Merchant, H., ed. (1999), *Yaraana: Gay Writing from India*. New Delhi: Penguin Books India (P) Ltd.

Mishra, K. M., trans. (1974), *Uttar Bharatmen Muslim Samaj* (in Hindi) [*Muslim Community in Northern India*]. Jaipur: Rajasthan Hindi Granth Akadami.

Nammalvar, N., Rao, A. V., Ramasubramaniam, C. (1983), Modification of homosexual behaviour: A case report. *Indian J. Clinical Psychology*, 10(1):35-38.

Nishant (1999), Poseur police. *Bombay Dost*, 6(4):11.

Patel, G., ed. & trans. (1984), *Kumarsambhava of Kalidasa*. Gandhinagar: Gujarat Sahitya Akademi.

Pradhan, P. V., Ayyar, K. S. & Bagadia, V. N. (1982a), Homosexuality: Treatment by behaviour modification. *Indian J. Psychiatry*, 24(1):80-83.

Pradhan, P. V., Ayyar, K. S. & Bagadia, V. N. (1982b), Male Homosexuality: A psychiatric study of thirteen cases. *Indian J. Psychiatry*, 24(2):182-186.

Rajat (1999), Coming out. *Bombay Dost*, 6(4):6.

Rangaswamy K. (1982), Difficulties in arousing and increasing heterosexual responsiveness in a homosexual. *Indian J. Clinical Psychology*, 9(2):147-151.

Ray, T., ed. & trans. (1944), *Ananga Ranga of Kalyanamalla*. Calcutta.

Samuel, M. (1990), Report of a seminar. *Bombay Dost*, 1(5):7.

Savaliya, M. L., ed. & trans. (2002), *Sharingar Shataka of Bhartruhari*, Third edition. Rajkot: Pravin Pustak Bhandar.

Shakuntala, D. (1977), *The World of Homosexuals*. New Delhi: Vikas Pub. House.

Shastri, D., trans. (1964), *Kama Sutra of Vatsyayana*. Varanasi: Chokhamba Sanskrit Series.

The Pioneer (2001), NHRC comes down on gay rights, August 2. Reprinted in *Pukaar*, 35, October 2001, p. 8.

Upadhyaya, S. C., ed. & trans. (1965), *Hindu Secrets of Love (Rati Rahasya of Kokkoka)*. Bombay: Taraporevala.

Vanita, R. & Kidwai, S., eds. (2000), *Same-Sex Love in India: Readings from Literature and History*. Delhi: MacMillan India Ltd. (and New York: St. Martin's Press).

Varma, P. (1979), *Sex Offences in India and Abroad: A Sociological Survey*. Delhi: B. R. Publishing Corporation.

Varma, R. M. (2000), The aftermath of social development: Challenges before psychiatry. *Commemorative Publication, Silver Jubilee of Annual Conference of Indian Psychiatric Society North Zone*, Delhi, pp. 24-33.

Yogi (1996), Ma, I am gay. *Bombay Dost*. 5(1):9-10.

The Emergence
of an International Lesbian, Gay,
and Bisexual Psychiatric Movement

Gene A. Nakajima, MD

SUMMARY. Since the 1990s, lesbian, gay and bisexual (LGB) psychiatrists have started to organize internationally. In particular, members of the Association of Gay and Lesbian Psychiatrists (AGLP), working collaboratively with the American Psychiatric Association (APA), have expanded their advocacy of LGB affirmative psychiatry outside of North America. Seven percent of AGLP is now comprised of international members. AGLP and APA have participated in efforts to depathologize homosexuality in Japan and China. Some progress has been made in increasing the awareness of LGB issues within the World Psychiatric Association (WPA). A future goal should be the elimination of stigmatising diagnoses like egodystonic sexual orientation from the ICD-10. *[Article copies available for a fee from The Haworth Document Delivery Service: 1-800-HAWORTH. E-mail address: <getinfo@haworthpressinc.com> Website: <http://www. HaworthPress.com> © 2003 by The Haworth Press, Inc. All rights reserved.]*

KEYWORDS. American Psychiatric Association, Association of Gay and Lesbian Psychiatrists, Ch\inese Classification of Mental Disorders, egodystonic sexual orientation, homosexuality, International Classification of Diseases, World Psychiatric Association

Gene A. Nakajima is Staff Psychiatrist, Center for Special Problems, San Francico, CA. Address correspondence to: Gene A. Nakajima, MD, Center for Special Problems, 1700 Jackson Street, San Francisco, CA 94109 (E-mail: Gnakajima@alumni.stanford.org).

The author thanks Howard Rubin, MD, Robert Cabaj, MD, Rochelle Klinger, MD, Richard Isay, MD, Jack Drescher, MD, Ellen Mercer, James Kent, MD, David Silven, PhD, Nico Hettinga, MD, Ken Hausman, and Herbert Sacks, MD for their assistance.

[Haworth co-indexing entry note]: "The Emergence of an International Lesbian, Gay, and Bisexual Psychiatric Movement." Nakajima, Gene A. Co-published simultaneously in *Journal of Gay & Lesbian Psychotherapy* (The Haworth Medical Press, an imprint of The Haworth Press, Inc.) Vol. 7, No. 1/2, 2003, pp. 165-188; and: *The Mental Health Professions and Homosexuality: International Perspectives* (ed: Vittorio Lingiardi, and Jack Drescher) The Haworth Medical Press, an imprint of The Haworth Press, Inc., 2003, pp. 165-188. Single or multiple copies of this article are available for a fee from The Haworth Document Delivery Service [1-800-HAWORTH, 9:00 a.m. - 5:00 p.m. (EST). E-mail address: getinfo@haworthpressinc.com].

10.1300/J236v07n01_10

ORGANIZATIONAL BACKGROUND

Because the Association of Gay and Lesbian Psychiatrists (AGLP) and the American Psychiatric Association (APA) have been instrumental in organizing lesbian-gay-bisexual (LGB) psychiatrists internationally, a brief description of these groups will follow. How United States (US) and Canadian psychiatrists struggled to establish formal structures will be described because these efforts are relevant to international attempts to organize LGB mental health professionals.

The APA is the world's largest psychiatric group with 37,000 members (American Psychiatric Association, n. d.). In 1973, it was the first major health organization to eliminate homosexuality as a mental illness (Monroe, 1974). AGLP was officially founded in 1985 as an organization independent of the APA. AGLP promotes its own positions on issues relating to homosexuality and has its own board, staff, and dues structure. With strong ties to the APA, AGLP serves as the organized voice of LGB professionals and patients in psychiatry in North America, and the organization currently has over 500 members (Haller, 2001).

AGLP traces its roots back to the late 1960s when LGB psychiatrists met at APA conventions and jokingly referred to themselves collectively as the "Gay PA" (Bayer, 1987). Eventually, this informal group evolved into the Caucus of Gay, Lesbian, and Bisexual (GLB) Members of the APA in the mid 1970s (Hire, 2001; Krajeski, 1996). While there is overlap between the AGLP and the APA's GLB Caucus, they are in fact separate groups. The GLB Caucus is regarded as a minority group within the APA, and as such has one vote in the APA Assembly (Drescher, 2002). In 1978, the Caucus petitioned the APA to create a Task Force on Gay, Lesbian, and Bisexual Issues; the task force was subsequently upgraded to a Committee of Gay, Lesbian and Bisexual (GLB) Issues in 1981. The charge of the APA committee on GLB Issues is to:

1. Investigate problems and issues which affect the mental health of the gay, lesbian and bisexual populations, such as stigmatization and discrimination;
2. Develop teaching programs to help correct the inadequate training of psychiatrists about homosexual issues;
3. Establish liaison with other [APA] components regarding homosexual issues; and
4. Promote the education of the APA membership and the general public about homosexuality (American Psychiatric Association, 2001, pp. D66-67).

In addition to its interest in GLB issues, the APA has an ongoing interest in international psychiatry and psychiatric issues. The Council of International

Affairs–now renamed the Commission on Global Psychiatry–is responsible for creating most official international positions for the APA. In the past, the APA had an independent Office of International Affairs, which employed two full time staff members.

INTERNATIONAL EFFORTS IN THE EARLY 1990S

AGLP celebrated its 20th anniversary in 1998. During its early history, the organization focused its efforts primarily on US concerns. In 1992, Richard Isay, MD chaired the APA's GLB Issues Committee. At an APA meeting, he attended a discussion about the World Psychiatric Association (WPA) and its upcoming World Congress of Psychiatry. The WPA is an international psychiatric association of representatives from national psychiatric groups. Currently, it is comprised of 115 affiliate member societies from 99 countries. Every three years it sponsors a World Congress during which resolutions are debated. Isay asked the APA to submit a resolution concerning homosexuality at the upcoming World Congress. This resolution was based upon an earlier landmark statement by APA on Homosexuality and Civil Rights, passed at the time when homosexuality was removed as a disorder from the *Diagnostic and Statistical Manual of Mental Disorders, Second Edition (DSM-II)* in 1973 (APA, 1968; APA, 1974).[1] In December 1992, the APA Board of Trustees passed the following resolution, which the APA delegate proposed and which the General Assembly of the WPA passed in June 1993 in Rio de Janeiro:

> Whereas homosexuality *per se* implies no impairment in judgment, stability, reliability, or general social or vocational capabilities, the WPA calls on its member organizations and individual members to urge the repeal of legislation that penalizes homosexual acts by consenting adults in private. And further, the WPA calls on these organizations and individuals to do all that is possible to decrease the stigma related to homosexuality wherever and whenever it may occur. (American Psychiatric Association Committee on Gay, Lesbian, and Bisexual Issues, 1993)

In December 1992, the APA Office of International Affairs–under the leadership of Ellen Mercer, a strong advocate for LGB issues–conducted a human rights survey of 125 psychiatric associations around the world. Thirty-four responded. The survey included three questions about homosexuality. Associations in 8 countries responded that the general feeling of their psychiatrists was that homosexuality was a mental illness. Eleven of the respondents stated that psychiatrists in their countries viewed homosexuality as deviant, even if homosexuality were no longer listed as a mental illness. Five of the responding societies did not believe that homosexuality was a mental illness or a deviation. The rest indicated that there was not a consensus about the issue in their country. Only 2 associations indicated that there were efforts in the psychiatric community to protect homosexual legal rights (Hausman, 1993). This survey pointed to the importance of educating psychiatrists worldwide that homosexuality is neither deviant nor an illness, and it demonstrated the need to encourage psychiatric associations to become involved in the civil rights of lesbian, gay and bisexual people.

In 1994, Mercer was working with an organization, the Geneva Initiative on Psychiatry, which disseminated education about human rights, including homosexuality. This organization collaborated with psychiatrists who had been isolated from international psychiatry before the fall of the Iron Curtain with the goal of reform in mental health in the former Soviet Union and Eastern/Central Europe. The Geneva Initiative produced a booklet concerning racism, sexism, and homophobia in psychiatry, which was published in several Eastern European languages, including Polish and Russian. Rochelle Klinger, MD, who succeeded Isay as chair of the APA Committee on GLB Issues, wrote an article for this booklet (Klinger, 1994).

DEPATHOLOGIZATION OF HOMOSEXUALITY IN JAPAN

Through a US graduate student specializing in Japanese history, I became acquainted with OCCUR, The Japan Association for the Lesbian and Gay Movement, a leading gay rights group. In the summer of 1994, OCCUR members traveled to the US to solicit support for their landmark anti-discrimination lawsuit against the city of Tokyo. I met with Masaki Inaba who was working to encourage the Japanese Society of Psychiatry and Neurology (JSPN) to adopt an explicitly affirmative policy toward homosexuality.

They published a pamphlet that included a brief description of their efforts to change psychiatric attitudes towards homosexuality. The pamphlet explained that, in general, homosexuality was considered a disease by Japanese psychiatrists, and that Japanese textbooks described homosexuality as deviant. OCCUR had unsuccessfully tried to meet with the JSPN to discuss this issue. In addition, they demanded that the JSPN publish an "official opinion" on homosexuality. They requested that members of the international psychiatric community write letters to the JSPN to ask them to depathologize homosexuality, and to contact their own psychiatric associations and have them contact the JSPN directly as well (OCCUR, 1994).

I sent OCCUR the recently passed 1993 WPA resolution encouraging member societies to decrease stigma about homosexuality, as well as the results of the above-mentioned APA survey of psychiatric associations and homosexuality which included the following response from the JSPN:

In Japan homosexuality up to now has evoked little public or professional interest and has not been discussed among psychiatrists. Psychiatrists are aware that homosexuality has been deleted from the disorder categories of *DSM* and *ICD*, but their opinion about the nature of homosexuality at this time is not known.

I felt the best way to assist OCCUR was to request the APA to ask the JSPN to endorse officially the World Health Organization (WHO) position that "sexual orientation by itself is not to be regarded as a disorder" as published in the *International Statistical Classification of Diseases and Health Related Problems, Tenth Revision, (ICD-10)* (World Health Organization, 1992b, p. 367). I contacted Mercer at the APA's International Affairs Office and drafted a letter for APA's medical director, Melvin Sabshin, MD (Nakajima, 1995). I also contacted Klinger and Terry Stein, MD, who was then a member of the APA Council on National Affairs, to request that APA take official action. In his letter, Sabshin indicated that the APA had deleted homosexuality as a disorder in 1973, and that ego-dystonic homosexuality was deleted in 1987. He also cited the 1993 WPA resolution. He ended the letter, urging:

> . . . the JSPN to join our [American Psychiatric] Association in making an official statement endorsing the *ICD-10* position that homosexuality is not a disorder. In addition, I urge the [Japanese] Society to adopt the WPA Statement. I also urge the Society to work with OCCUR and other such groups to decrease the stigma of homosexuality in Japan. (personal communication, October 13, 1994, Letter to Board of Directors, JSPN)

Masahiro Asai, MD, the president of the JSPN replied. He said the JSPN had recently endorsed ICD-10's position:

> Concerning the official classification of diseases, the Japanese Government and the Ministry of Health and Welfare adopted *ICD-10* as the official statistical classification of illness, injury and cause of death on and after the January 1st of this year 1995. *ICD-10* had [been] translated into Japanese and officially published. *ICD-10* "F66 Psychological and behavioral disorders associated with sexual development and orientation" has a note: "Sexual orientation by itself is not to be regarded as a disorder." This sentence is translated into Japanese literally and included in the official Japanese classification.

> We esteem *ICD-10* as the official Japanese classification and are learning many things from *ICD-10*.

I hope [for] future good relationship between the APA and the JSPN. (personal communication, January 23, 1995, Letter to Sabshin)[2]

DEPATHOLOGIZATION OF HOMOSEXUALITY IN CHINA

In the fall of 1997, I read an article about Wan Yan Hai, who was a visiting scholar at the University of Southern California. He was working to delete homosexuality as a mental disorder in China (Yanhai, 2001). At our first meeting, he informed me that the *Chinese Classification of Mental Disorder-Second Revision (CCMD 2-R)* acknowledged that homosexuality had been depathologized in the international classification, but it clearly stated that Chinese psychiatry did not follow those changes (Wah-shan, 2000; Lee, 1996; Chinese Society of Psychiatry (CSP) of the Chinese Medical Association, 1995). I again contacted Mercer from the APA Office of International Affairs to request that a letter to the CSP task force revising the *CCMD* be sent. Robert Cabaj, MD, a former AGLP president, also spoke to Sabshin, about contacting the *CCMD* task force. Coincidentally, Mercer was working on a joint meeting between officers of the CSP and the APA at a regional meeting of the WPA in Beijing in October 1997. She asked the President of the APA at the time, Herbert Sacks, MD, to mention to the CSP the importance of deleting homosexuality as a mental illness. Although he gave a plenary talk at the conference, he brought up the subject of homosexuality in the context of other human rights abuses in private meetings (H. S. Sacks, personal communication, March 30, 2002; Nakajima, 2001; Sacks, 1997). To contact AGLP members for their help and advice, I also helped Yan Hai write an article about the situation for the *Newsletter of AGLP* (Yanhai, 1997).

In March 2001, the CSP announced that it would eliminate homosexuality as a mental disorder in *CCMD-3* (Lee, 2001). However, they decided to add ego-dystonic homosexuality (Chinese Society of Psychiatry, 2001).[3] Although it is unknown how much influence the APA had in this decision, the *CCMD* task force acknowledged the APA's encouragement to change the classification (Chu, 2001). The Chinese Society for the Study of Sexual Minorities also mentioned that the CSP sent members to attend the APA annual meeting in 2000 to solicit advice. The vice president of CSP, Chen Yanfang, MD, in announcing the change, stated that it brought China closer to the WHO and the APA positions (Chinese Society for the Study of Sexual Minorities, 2001). The task force also conducted a field study examining 51 gay men and found that their data did not support the continued inclusion of homosexuality as a mental disorder because only 6 had emotional problems (Mental Disorder Redefined, 2001; Wu, 2003). In both Japan and China, pressure from US psychiatry was helpful in efforts to depathologize homosexuality.

WORLD PSYCHIATRIC ASSOCIATION (WPA)

Building on the work of Isay and the 1993 WPA resolution, I organized the first symposium on lesbian and gay issues at a World Congress of Psychiatry with Guy Glass, MD of New York and Siegmund Dannecker, MD of Berlin. Ulrich Gooss, MD, a psychiatrist from Frankfurt, and a co-chair of the German Federation of Gays in the Health Service (*Bundesarbeits Gemeinschaft Schwule im Gesundheitswesen* (BASG)), had attended the World Congress in Rio de Janeiro in 1993, and reported that there had been no lesbian-gay presentations. Through announcements in the *Newsletter of the AGLP* and at the 1995 Miami APA annual meeting, seven speakers were chosen for a symposium entitled *Perspectives on Gay Affirmative Psychiatry* for the Tenth World Congress in Madrid in August 1996 (Glass et al., 1996).

Glass introduced the symposium with "An overview of Gay Affirmative Psychiatry." I presented on "Developing Gay Asian Identities in Confucian Cultures" while Francisco González, MD, a Cuban-American psychiatrist spoke on "Homophobic Stigma and Culture" (Nakajima, 1996). Olli Stålström described the rise of sexual conversion or "reparative" therapy in Finland. Howard Rubin, MD spoke about the depiction of homosexuality in US psychiatric textbooks, focusing on changes in various editions of Kaplan and Sadock's textbook. Jürgen Graffe, MD presented a study in which he had interviewed directors of psychoanalytic institutes in West Germany about admission of gay applicants (Stakelbeck and Frank, 2003). Mercer gave an overview of the APA resolutions and policies adopted by a number of international organizations concerning homosexuality. Sabshin, then the APA medical director and a member of the executive committee of the WPA, was the most prominent discussant. Because of his presence, many APA and WPA officials came to the symposium, and it was covered in the APA newspaper, *Psychiatric News* (Hausman, 1996). One of the leading national daily newspapers of Spain, *El Mundo*, covered the symposium as well (Velasco, 1996). Most important, for many of the international psychiatrists, it represented their first symposium devoted to lesbian-gay issues at a psychiatric meeting.

In Madrid, BASG and AGLP co-sponsored a networking meeting for lesbian, gay and bisexual psychiatrists. The process of obtaining a room from the WPA (greatly facilitated by Mercer) required over a year of effort including several faxes and phone calls. A couple of months before the meeting, we were suddenly informed that the APA was required to request a room from the secretary of the WPA. After this letter was sent, we were granted a room at the last moment. Several signs about the meeting were posted throughout the convention center; however, they needed to be replenished because they were torn down repeatedly. At the beginning of the meeting, two people from the company contracted to organize the conference barged in and demanded to know how we had obtained the room. Unfortunately, the final details were done by phone and we did not have written confirmation. Mercer took charge, presented her business card to the two people, and we proceeded with the meeting.

Over 40 psychiatrists from 20 countries attended, including Canada, Finland, the Dominican Republic, Switzerland, Germany, Poland, Spain, the Czech Republic, Chile, Argentina, United Kingdom, South Africa, Brazil, Mexico, Italy, Norway, the Netherlands, Sweden, the US, and France (Glass, 1996). Participants introduced themselves and spoke briefly about their experiences as gay psychiatrists in their countries. For many, it was the first opportunity to talk with LGB colleagues in a professional meeting. Because a large number of people from Spain did not understand English well, AGLP members, Ken Campos, MD and González translated. Prior to the meeting, we discovered an advertisement for a practice of psychologists and psychiatrists called *Grupo Les-Hom, Servicios Psicológicos Para la Poblácion Gai y Lesbiana* in a Madrid gay newspaper. We contacted them, and they too attended the meeting. They subsequently arranged two informal dinners at local lesbian-gay restaurants, which facilitated further networking.

Given the difficulty obtaining a meeting room and in an effort to provide a mechanism for psychiatrists to organize internationally, it was decided to explore the establishment of a formal section of LGB issues in the WPA. Mercer provided us with the information to start a section. Initially, we needed ten psychiatrists (no more than two from a single country) to start an ad hoc section, which would then require approval by the WPA's executive committee and subsequently the General Assembly at the next World Congress (World Psychiatric Association, 2000). We easily obtained the ten psychiatrists at the 1997 APA meeting, and Dannecker sent the request.

Ahmed Okasha, MD of Cairo, the WPA Secretary of Sections, wrote back that the executive committee had denied our request in their April 1998 meeting in Beirut (personal communication, Letter to Dannecker, April 20, 1998). The committee had also received a request to start a section on Human Sexuality, and he suggested that this section could accommodate our needs. Dannecker wrote back asking the executive committee to reconsider. We discovered that the original request had been to establish a section on Sexual Disorders and that the executive committee had broadened its compass to Human Sexuality. We wrote:

> . . . Gay and lesbian concerns are not related to sexual disorders and their treatments. To associate our group with sexual behavior in this way would be a fundamental mistake that would send quite the wrong message to professionals and their patients around the world.
>
> Most psychiatrists who are interested in Lesbian, Gay, and Bisexual Issues would assume quite rightly that "human sexuality" mostly deals

with sexual disorders and their treatments, and only peripherally involves lesbian, gay, and bisexual issues. One of the important functions
of a Lesbian, Gay, and Bisexual Issues section is to make it easier for
psychiatrists interested in those issues to meet and exchange ideas from
their home countries. We do not think that this coming together will happen in a Human Sexuality Section, which will have many different areas
of focus.

Gay and lesbian issues are akin to those of a cultural group. Sexuality
is only one part of the conception of what it is to be gay or lesbian. To focus on sexuality would be to propagate the stereotype that gays and lesbians can be completely defined by sexual behavior. The principal need for
this section is to provide a forum in which minority issues can be addressed, such as discrimination, homophobia in psychiatric training, and
gay affirmative therapies. We cannot underestimate the importance of
examining homophobia as a serious cause of affective disorders including depression and suicide, youth suicide, substance abuse, and its role in
personality disorders. (Personal communication, Letter from Dannecker
to Okasha, May 1998)

Dannecker and I also informally met with Okasha at the Toronto APA
meeting in May 1998. We felt that he would not be sympathetic to our request
for starting a section, and we were not surprised when he wrote back that the
executive committee met again in Johannesburg and declined our second request:

... We reviewed with great care and concern your proposal to create a
section of Lesbian, Gay, and Bisexual Issues in Psychiatry. The Executive Committee found that the scientific objectives overlap with the new
ad-hoc Section entitled "Psychiatry and Human Sexuality" and your participation in this existing section will enrich the scope of the section.

The other issues you mentioned in your proposal such as depression,
substance abuse, and suicide can be dealt with in the respective sections. . . .

As to the problem of discrimination, the Ethics Committee of the
WPA is preparing some specific guidelines, one being on ethnic discrimination, but this can be extended in this Committee or the next to include
ethical guidelines for discrimination because of sexual inclinations.

Enclosed you will find a copy of the letter sent by Professor Norman
Sartorius,[4] President of the WPA, to Dr. Hubschmid, President of
the Swiss Psychiatric Association. (Personal communication, Letter to
Dannecker, September 21, 1998)

Because of the rejection of our request for a section, we have decided to work with the Human Sexuality Section until we can start one of our own. Rubén Hernández-Serrano, MD from Caracas, the former President of the International Association of Sexology, who had proposed the new Human Sexuality Section, became its head. He knew Carlos Greaves, MD, a Venezuelan American psychiatrist from Palo Alto, CA, and an active AGLP member. We invited Hernández-Serrano to come to an AGLP meeting for international participants, which Greaves also attended, at the 1999 APA meeting in Washington, DC. Greaves and I subsequently attended the meeting of the Human Sexuality Section at the WPA Congress in Hamburg and are currently members. To show our willingness to collaborate with Hernández-Serrano, I participated in a symposium that the Human Sexuality section organized in Hamburg, and spoke on the prevalence and treatment of sexual dysfunction in a study of 200 Asian and Pacific Islanders with HIV/AIDS in the US.

International conferences typically require a long period to review proposals for presentations, but the abstract submission deadline for the August 1999 Eleventh World Congress in Hamburg was unusually early–16 months before the conference. Because of several deadline extensions, we were able to organize 43 presenters of 69 abstracts into 16 symposiums. This large number of submissions appeared to disturb conference organizers. They rejected several of the symposia and asked that many be combined. By March 1999, only three symposia had been accepted, and several had neither been accepted nor rejected. Because of the large number of rejections, Dannecker and I met informally with the vice-chair of the scientific committee of the Hamburg conference, Wolfgang Gaebel, MD at the 1999 APA annual meeting. We gave him information about AGLP presentations, and he told us he had noticed how gay and lesbian topics had been integrated into the APA annual meeting. Eventually, six symposia were accepted with 26 speakers (World Congress of Psychiatry, 1999).

In Hamburg, LGB activities were expanded. Dannecker, with the help of BASG, organized a reception at the Magnus Hirschfeld Zentrum, Hamburg's lesbian and gay community center.[5] Over 75 people attended the reception funded by the Solvay pharmaceutical company. We organized two informal dinners, and rented rooms at a gay-lesbian hotel in Hamburg, where Cabaj led an informal discussion group on coming out as a gay psychiatrist, and Julie Leavitt, MD led one for lesbian participants.

The conference provided free booths for non-profit organizations like AGLP. Several hundred psychiatrists saw the booth, many visited, took copies of the *Newsletter of the AGLP* and membership brochures, browsed through books and samples of the *Journal of Gay & Lesbian Psychotherapy*. Some discussed issues about homosexuality in their countries. We also provided copies of the APA's *Fact Sheet: Gay, Lesbian, and Bisexual Issues,* which summarized official APA positions (American Psychiatric Association, 2000a).

Cabaj held a signing for his *Textbook of Homosexuality and Mental Health* (Cabaj and Stein, 1996). A LGB organizational meeting sponsored by the Human Sexuality Section was arranged. The affiliation with a WPA section greatly facilitated this room request. During the meeting, a discussion was held on whether to start an international LGB psychiatry organization, but there was insufficient interest. However, attendees expressed interest in an Internet discussion list serve, which we hope to start soon.

Based on the work I had done with China and Japan, I felt that the issue of depathologizing homosexuality was an important one to press. I believed an official WPA position would be useful in countries like China whose psychiatric society, at the time of the conference, still considered homosexuality a mental disorder. I wanted to introduce a non-controversial resolution, which endorsed the *ICD-10* stand depathologizing homosexuality. I assumed that it would be easy to pass since the WHO had already approved depathologization. The resolution stated:

> Whereas in 1992, on the basis of large body of scientific research, the WHO deleted homosexuality as a disorder in the *ICD-10*, stating "sexual orientation by itself is not be regarded as a disorder," the WPA calls on its member organizations and individual members to urge the elimination of homosexuality as a disorder in all medical and psychiatric textbooks and other nosologic systems. And further, the WPA calls on these organizations and individuals to do all that is possible to oppose any mental health evaluation or treatment which is based upon the assumption that homosexuality *per se* is a mental disorder.

This resolution was discussed at a conference call of the APA Council of International Affairs. It passed easily thanks to the help of Lawrence Hartmann, MD, a member of the Council and the first openly gay president of the APA. This resolution was the only one that the APA submitted for consideration at the WPA Hamburg meeting. Usually, the APA president is the US delegate for the WPA; however, this resolution was scheduled last for discussion in the General Assembly. Because it was brought up after midnight, the APA president at the time, Allan Tasman, MD, asked the immediate past president, Harold Eist, MD, to stay for the debate. Unfortunately the WPA failed to make a decision about the resolution after more than 30 minutes of discussion (Nakajima, 1999). Instead, the WPA Executive Committee is supposed to discuss this resolution and reintroduce it at the next General Assembly in Yokohama in August 2002. Ruedi Gloor, MD reports that since Hamburg, the WPA president has received positive input from representatives of some psychiatric associations, including the president of the Swiss Psychiatric Association, Tedy

Hubschmid, MD (personal communication, March 15, 2000, Letter from Hubschmid to Okasha).

After Hamburg, AGLP organized a symposium and prepared a booth for a smaller conference in Paris in June 2000 celebrating the Jubilee (50th anniversary of the founding) of the WPA (Nakajima et al., 2000). At this meeting, I met informally with Eist who told me that he had strongly advocated for the resolution in Hamburg. However, the delegate from the United Kingdom during the debate asked how could it be certain that homosexuality is not a mental illness. Other delegates then expressed reservations about the resolution, and it was tabled. Eist, who is currently chair of the APA Commission on Global Affairs, has been asked by the WPA to be a consultant on this issue. Hopefully, this resolution will be brought up and passed without significant change at the Yokohama meeting. Soliciting national psychiatric associations to support the resolution will be important.

STARTING AN AGLP INTERNATIONAL COMMITTEE

In anticipation of the Madrid WPA Congress, Kenn Ashley, MD and I planned a meeting of international psychiatrists attending the 1996 New York APA annual meeting. The APA annual meetings are the world's largest psychiatric conferences, and increasing numbers of international psychiatrists attend; 5,186 (33%) of the 15,949 who registered for the 2001 conference in New Orleans lived outside the US and Canada (Annual Meeting, 2001). Although international psychiatrists have attended LGB functions at the APA meeting, particularly workshops and symposia which were part of the official APA program, they rarely participated in most AGLP events. Major functions like the opening reception with more than 300 people made many feel "lost." Most North American psychiatrists attending AGLP functions generally spent time with colleagues from current or past workplaces or with acquaintances from past AGLP functions. International psychiatrists often did not know many people at AGLP functions and did not feel included because they had not attended APA meetings regularly. Few psychiatrists outside North America joined AGLP, because of its primary focus on the APA annual meeting. Most international psychiatrists found out about AGLP events through posters or the information booth at the convention center. They discovered AGLP events late in the conference, missing many functions like the Saturday pre-convention symposium, the Sunday evening opening reception, or the closing dinner and awards ceremony on Wednesday, which required early reservations. By establishing a meeting time for international psychiatrists and interested North American AGLP members, we wanted to help them feel more welcome in AGLP. We placed notices about the meeting in the *Daily Bulletin*, an informational newspaper available at the annual APA meeting. We also placed signs in the International Hospitality Center, again with the assistance of Mercer. The meeting was listed in the *Newsletter of the AGLP* and the AGLP booklet listing LGB events at the conference.

At the first meeting, which took place in the AGLP hospitality suite, 12 international psychiatrists attended. Mercer answered questions about how to become an international member of the APA, which, among other benefits, reduces the annual meeting registration fee.[6] An international psychiatrist who wanted to join the APA in the past needed three reference letters from APA members, which were usually difficult to obtain.[7] By writing letters of reference, AGLP members have helped several international psychiatrists become APA members. At the meeting, we answered questions about AGLP, and international psychiatrists discussed the situation for LGB psychiatrists in their own countries.

For several years, AGLP had held a reception for LGB psychiatrists of color including Asian Pacific Islanders, African Americans, Latino/as, and other minority psychiatrists. In New York, we added international psychiatrists to this reception. We have continued to organize meetings and receptions for international psychiatrists, and these efforts have tremendously increased their participation at all AGLP events. For example, at the 2001 New Orleans APA meeting, over 40 international psychiatrists attended the international-minority AGLP reception, which was followed by a dinner. A reduced international rate for AGLP[8] was introduced because most international psychiatrists did not attend APA meetings frequently. International members now account for seven percent of AGLP (Haller, 2001). Ashley and I currently chair a newly formed AGLP International Committee.

At the 1996 New York APA meeting, German and Dutch psychiatrists, who met at an AGLP symposium, planned and presented a workshop for the following year in San Diego called *Gay and Lesbian Psychiatrists: A European Perspective* (Dannecker et al., 1997). Proposing workshops is challenging for international participants because the deadline for submission is in September of the year before the May conference. In contrast to the US, where American Medical Association (1991) ethics guidelines do not allow physicians to accept paid trips from pharmaceutical companies, other countries do not restrict companies from providing support for psychiatrists to attend meetings. Because of financial constraints, many international psychiatrists will attend conferences only if they are sponsored, and they frequently do not find out about sponsorship until significantly after abstract submission deadlines. At the Toronto APA meeting, I organized another workshop by international psychiatrists, which included psychiatrists from Norway and Switzerland, titled *International Perspectives on Gay Psychiatry* (Nakajima et al. 1998). Dutch gay psychiatrists have presented two workshops at annual meetings, one called

Gay Psychiatrists: An Amsterdam Perspective (Hettinga et al., 1998) and the other *Narcissism Below Sea Level: A Dutch View of Future Gay Developments* (Hettinga et al., 2001).

AGLP sponsors pre-conference symposia on the Saturday before the APA annual meeting. At the 1997 San Diego meeting, Nico Hettinga, MD gave a presentation titled "International Fears and National Affairs: Same-Sex Marriage in the Netherlands." This paper was subsequently published in the *Newsletter of the AGLP*, the first article written by an international psychiatrist (Hettinga, 1998). International psychiatrists have helped AGLP members learn about mental health issues in other countries. Interestingly, most international psychiatrists who have presented at APA meetings except for the Dutch have not presented at their own psychiatric societies.

AGLP members have been active internationally outside the WPA. Terry Stein, MD presented a paper about eliminating ego-dystonic homosexuality from DSM-III-R at a conference sponsored by the International Gay and Lesbian Association and the University of Utrecht, in the Netherlands in 1987 called "Homosexuality beyond Disease." Isay, after the publication of his book *Being Homosexual: Gay Men and Their Development* (1989), travelled to several European countries to lecture. His book has had several European printings and has been translated into several European languages (Stakelbeck and Frank, 2003). Kewchang Lee, MD presented a paper on Gay Asian Americans at the Seventh Scientific Meeting of the Pacific Rim College of Psychiatrists in Fukuoka, Japan (Lee, 1995). The Australian Gay, Lesbian, and Bisexual Interest Group in Psychiatry organizes a yearly conference which coincides with the Sydney Gay and Lesbian Mardi Gras (see Appendix for contact information). Cabaj presented at the third annual conference in 1997 and the fifth in 1999, while Ashley, Glass, and I presented at the fourth annual conference (Glass, 1998).[9] Michael King, MD, President of the Section of Psychiatry from the Royal Society of Medicine organized a conference on Gay and Lesbian Mental Health in London in October 1997, at which Rubin and Isay presented papers (Gosling, 1998). King has subsequently started a Gay and Lesbian Mental Health Interest Group in the Royal College of Psychiatrists.[10] To start an ongoing collaboration between the two groups, AGLP members Cabaj and Ronald Hellman, MD participated in a workshop with King at the Royal College of Psychiatrists' annual meeting in Cardiff, Wales in June, 2002.

APA resolutions about homosexuality, largely crafted by its Gay, Lesbian, and Bisexual Issues Committee have been used internationally. For example, Reidar Kjaer, MD and colleagues used the APA resolutions against sexual conversion or "reparative" therapy to write a similar one which was adopted by the Norwegian Psychiatric Association (Kjaer, 2003; Kjaer and Selle, 2001; APA Committee on Gay, Lesbian, and Bisexual Issues, 1999; American Psychiatric Association, 2000b). Jack Drescher, MD, current chair of the APA Committee on Gay, Lesbian, and Bisexual Issues was contacted by Stålström because a Finnish member of Parliament was making arguments on the efficacy of conversion-"reparative" therapy, during debates on a proposed domestic partnership law. Drescher provided the Finnish government with the APA resolutions rejecting conversion-"reparative" therapy as well as the recent APA resolution endorsing same-sex unions (Hausman, 2001; Olarte, 2001; American Psychiatric Association Trustees, 2001).

Ralph Roughton, MD, the former Chair of the Committee on Issues of Homosexuality of the American Psychoanalytic Association and an AGLP member, was appointed to the House of Delegates of the International Psychoanalytic Association. He has been leading efforts to ensure non-discrimination for LGB applicants to psychoanalytic institutes worldwide (Roughton, 2003).

FUTURE GOALS

AGLP's executive board and executive director have been extremely supportive of recent efforts to expand internationally. More psychiatrists outside North America are continuing to join AGLP and participate in its activities. Since the APA meetings attract so many international participants, integrating their needs into AGLP remains an important, ongoing task.

Much of what was accomplished in the past few years was made possible through strong advocacy from the APA.[11] The International Affairs Office has been eliminated, and many of its functions have been subsumed under International Research Programs in the DSM Programs of the Division of Research (Tasman, 2000). In the future, the APA may not be as capable of proactive advocacy on LGB issues in international psychiatry because there may be less institutional support to do the work.

Although the WPA has not been open to formal recognition of LGB psychiatrists, continuing to work within the WPA structure is important. Many LGB psychiatrists attend their conferences and organize meetings and symposia. There are no other worldwide psychiatric meetings which leaders of national psychiatric associations regularly attend.

Although the resolution submitted by the APA in Hamburg was not voted on, a discussion of this issue among the delegates and their national psychiatric associations on how to vote in Yokohama is now in progress. At the time of this writing, we have begun preparation for the Twelfth World Psychiatric Congress in Yokohama in August 2002, and we are working with OCCUR, the Japanese activist group. Three lesbian-gay symposiums and workshops have been accepted. The Thirteenth World Psychiatric Congress will be in Cairo, September 10-15, 2005, and the Fourteenth will be in Prague in 2008. Two smaller meetings, International Congresses of the WPA, are tentatively scheduled for June 18-21, 2003 in Vienna, and November 10-13, 2004 in Florence and a regional conference in Caracas in for October 2-4, 2003 (WPA, 2002). A lesbian-gay-bisexual presence will be important at all those, as well as in regional WPA conferences. Hopefully, the current resolution will be passed and the WPA executive committee will reconsider starting a LGB section. Having such a section will be important until more interest is generated in starting an independent international LGB psychiatric organization.

In the event the WPA votes to endorse *ICD-10's* position depathologizing homosexuality, working with the WPA on eliminating problematic diagnoses in the *ICD-10* inconsistent with *DSM* could be a future goal. Although the WHO deleted homosexuality as a mental disorder in *ICD-10*, it included the diagnosis of "Egodystonic [sic] sexual orientation." In the previous edition, *ICD-9*, homosexuality was listed under Sexual Deviations and Disorders, with the statement "Exclusive or predominant sexual attraction for person of the same sex with or without physical relationship. Code homosexuality here whether or not it is considered a mental disorder" (World Health Organization, 1977, p. 196). According to the *ICD-10, April, 1988 Draft*, the WHO, although eliminating homosexuality, considered adding three diagnoses: ego-dystonic sexual orientation associated with heterosexuality (Code F66.1); ego-dystonic sexual orientation associated with homosexuality (Code F66.2), and ego-dystonic sexual orientation associated with bisexuality (Code F66.3) (Junge, 1989; World Health Organization, 1988). Eventually, the WHO modified these three diagnoses into one, Egodystonic Sexual Orientation (Code F66.1), in the main *ICD-10* volume that was published. The *ICD-10* defines Egodystonic sexual orientation as "The gender identity or sexual preference (heterosexual, homosexual, bisexual, or prepubertal) is not in doubt, but the individual wishes it were different because of associated psychological and behavioural disorders, and may seek treatment in order to change it."

The *ICD-10* has two other problematic diagnoses. One is Sexual Maturation Disorder (Code F66.0):

> The patient suffers from uncertainty about his or her gender identity or sexual orientation, which causes anxiety or depression. Most commonly this occurs in adolescents who are not certain whether they are homosexual, heterosexual, or bisexual in orientation, or in individuals who, after a period of apparently stable sexual orientation (often within a longstanding relationship), find that their sexual orientation is changing.

The other problematic diagnosis is Sexual Relationship Disorder (Code F66.2): "The gender identity or sexual orientation (heterosexual, homosexual, or bisexual) is responsible for difficulties in forming or maintaining a relationship with a sexual partner (World Health Organization, 1992b, pp. 367-8)." A supplementary *ICD-10* volume, published on *Mental and Behavioral Disorders with Clinical descriptions and diagnostic guidelines,* suggests that the F66 diagnoses can be further subdivided more precisely by recording the sexual orientation with a fifth character code (Heterosexual (F66.x0), Homosexual (F66.x1), Bisexual (F66.x2), or Other, including prepubertal (F66.x8)) (World Health Organization, 1992a, p. 221; Drimmelen-Krabbe et al., 1994). Therefore, someone hypothetically with "Egodystonic sexual orientation, Homosexual" would be coded as F66.11. Of great concern is that unethical practitioners advocating for sexual conversion or "reparative" therapy may misuse these three diagnoses.[12]

In the future, when committees form to consider *ICD-11,* elimination of Egodystonic Sexual Orientation, Sexual Maturation Disorder, and Sexual Relationship Disorder could be a goal for LGB psychiatrists worldwide. Having an international network of LGB psychiatrists could be instrumental in working with the WHO, WPA, and delegates to the *ICD-11* committees. As a start, national psychiatric associations calling for the deletion of these diagnoses could pass their own resolutions. AGLP will need to work with the International Research Programs of the *DSM* Programs in the APA Office of Research to have the APA use its influence in the WHO to resolve favorably this major discrepancy between *ICD* and *DSM.*

Although a worldwide movement for LGB psychiatry has started, very few countries have formal or informal groups. Only the United Kingdom and US have formal groups within their national psychiatric associations. Some countries are starting to organize; for example, in Australia lectures and informal dinners have taken place at the Royal Australian and New Zealand College of Psychiatrists conventions. Canada (through AGLP), the US, and Australia have independent LGB psychiatry organizations. Hopefully in the future, more countries will formalize LGB psychiatry committees within their national psychiatry groups, which will ultimately strengthen international LGB psychiatry. With greater organization, goals, like education about LGB issues in psychiatry and the elimination of pathologizing diagnoses can be achieved.

NOTES

1. Whereas, homosexuality *per se* implies no impairment in judgment, stability, reliability, or general social or vocational capabilities, therefore, be it resolved that the APA deplores all public and private discrimination against homosexuals in such areas as employment, housing, public accommodation, and licensing, and declares that no burden of proof of such judgment, capacity, or reliability shall be placed upon homosexuals greater than that imposed on other persons. Further the [APA] supports and urges the enactment of civil rights legislation at the local, state, and federal level that

would offer homosexual citizens the same protection now guaranteed to others on the basis of race, creed, color, etc. Further the [APA] supports and urges the repeal of all discriminatory legislation singling out homosexual acts by consenting adults in private.

2. JSPN sent this letter directly to the APA; OCCUR was somewhat upset because they found out about the change through their contacts with the APA. OCCUR has subsequently used this letter to increase awareness that the Japanese medical establishment officially no longer considered homosexuality a mental illness (Summerhawk, McMahill, & McDonald, 1998).

3. This action was similar to the APA's, which deleted homosexuality in 1973, but then added ego-dystonic homosexuality to *DSM-III* (American Psychiatric Association, 1980). See Bayer, 1987.

4. The letter from Sartorius was in response to a letter from the president of the Swiss Psychiatric Association, probably the only WPA member society that wrote a letter specifically supporting the section.

5. Named for the physician-sexologist who started the first gay rights group in 1897 (Stakelbeck & Frank, 2003).

6. Currently, International APA Membership is $150 a year; it reduces registration fee for the annual meeting by $210.

7. Now only one letter is needed.

8. Now $60, compared to $185 for US and Canadian members.

9. In 2001, the conference was not held in Sydney but in Melbourne. In November 2002, the group will host an additional conference coinciding with Gay Games.

10. It took King several years to secure 120 Royal College of Psychiatrists members willing to become members of the section (see Appendix).

11. Melvin Sabshin, MD, as APA medical director, had been a strong advocate for LGB issues as well as for US involvement in international psychiatry. Ellen Mercer, as head of the International Affairs Office, took a proactive stance on LGB issues. Unfortunately, Sabshin has retired from his position and Mercer has also left the APA.

12. The *ICD* situation parallels the earlier one with the *DSM*. When homosexuality was eliminated as a diagnosis in 1973, the APA added "sexual orientation disturbance" until Ego-dystonic Homosexuality was added in *DSM-III* (APA, 1980). Subsequently, in 1987, Ego-dystonic Homosexuality was eliminated in *DSM-III-R*, because very few people used the diagnosis, and no research or empirical data supported its continuation (Bayer, 1987; Krajeski, 1996; American Psychiatric Association, 1987).

REFERENCES

American Medical Association (1991), Gifts to physicians from industry. *JAMA*, 265:501.

American Psychiatric Association (1968), *Diagnostic and Statistical Manual of Mental Disorders, 2nd edition*. Washington, DC: American Psychiatric Press.

American Psychiatric Association (1974), Position statement on homosexuality and civil rights. *Amer. J. Psychiat.*, 131:497.

American Psychiatric Association (1980), *Diagnostic and Statistical Manual of Mental Disorders, 3rd edition*. Washington, DC: American Psychiatric Press.

American Psychiatric Association (1987), *Diagnostic and Statistical Manual of Mental Disorders, 3rd edition-Revised*. Washington, DC: American Psychiatric Press.

American Psychiatric Association (2000a), *Fact Sheet: Gay, Lesbian, and Bisexual Issues*. Retrieved March 30, 2002, from <http://www.psych.org/public_info/gaylesbianbisexualissues22701.pdf>.

American Psychiatric Association (2000b), Commission on Psychotherapy by Psychiatrists (COPP): Position statement on therapies focused on attempts to change sexual orientation (Reparative or conversion therapies). *Amer. J. Psychiat.*, (157):1719-1721.

American Psychiatric Association (2001), *Operations Manual of the Board of Trustees of the American Psychiatric Association*. Retrieved March 29, 2002, from <http://www.psych.org/governance/operationsmanual.pdf>.

American Psychiatric Association (n. d.), *About APA*. Retrieved March 30, 2002, from <http://www.psych.org/aboutapa.cfm>.

American Psychiatric Association Committee on Gay, Lesbian, and Bisexual Issues (1993), Position statement on homosexuality. *Amer. J. Psychiat.*, 150:686.

American Psychiatric Association Committee on Gay, Lesbian, and Bisexual Issues (1999), Position statement on psychiatric treatment and sexual orientation. *Amer. J. Psychiat.*, 156:1131.

Annual Meeting Continues to Garner Rave Reviews (2001), *Psychiatric News*, 36(16):17, August 17. Retrieved March 20, 2002, from <http://pn.psychiatryonline.org/cgi/content/full/36/16/17>.

APA Trustees Take Action on Carveouts, Other Major Issues (2001), *Psychiatric News*, 36(1):1, January 5. Retrieved March 30, 2002, from American Psychiatric Association Web Site: <http://www.psych.org/pnews/01-01-05/trustees.html>.

Bayer, R. (1987), *Homosexuality and American Psychiatry*. Second edition. Princeton, NJ: Princeton University Press.

Cabaj, R. P. & Stein, T. S., eds. (1996), *Textbook of Homosexuality and Mental Health*. Washington, DC: American Psychiatric Press.

Chinese Society for the Studies of Sexual Minorities (2001), *Homosexuality Depathologized in China*. Retrieved March 30, 2002, from <http://www.csssm.org/English/e7htm>.

Chinese Society of Psychiatry of the Chinese Medical Association (1995), *Chinese Classification of Mental Disorders, Second Edition, Revised (CCMD-2-R)*. Nanjing, China: Dong Nan University Press.

Chinese Society of Psychiatry (2001), *Chinese Classification of Mental Disorders Third Edition (CCMD-3)*. Shandong, China: Shandong Publishing House of Science and Technology.

Chu, H. (2001), Chinese psychiatrists decide homosexuality isn't abnormal. *Los Angeles Times*, March 15.

Dannecker, S., Graffe, J., Hettinga, N. F. & Oele S. (1997), *Gay and Lesbian Psychiatrists: A European Perspective*. Workshop conducted at the 150th Annual Meeting of the American Psychiatric Association, San Diego, CA, May.

Drescher, J. (2002), An interview with Edward Hanin, MD. *J. Gay & Lesb. Psychother.*, 6(2):87-97.

Drimmelen-Krabbe, J. J. van, Ustun, T. B., Thompson, D. H., l'Hours, A., Orley, J. & Sartorius, N. (1994), Homosexuality in the *International Classification of Diseases*: A clarification [Letter to the editor]. *JAMA*, 272:1660.

Glass, G. (1996), Editor's column. *Newsletter of the Association of Gay and Lesbian Psychiatrists*, 22(4): 2,10-11, December.

Glass, G. (1998), Editor's column. *Newsletter of the Association of Gay and Lesbian Psychiatrists*, 24(2):2, April.

Glass, G., Dannecker, S., Nakajima, G. A., Rubin, H. C., González, F., Stålström, O., Graffe J., Mercer, E. & Sabshin, M. (1996), *Perspectives on Gay Affirmative Psychiatry*. Symposium conducted at the Tenth World Congress of Psychiatry, Madrid, Spain, August.

Gosling J. (1998), Gay and lesbian mental health conference in London. *Newsletter of the Association of Gay and Lesbian Psychiatrists*, 24(1):15, January.

Haller, E. (2001), AGLP Fall Business Meeting. *Newsletter of the Association of Gay and Lesbian Psychiatrists*, 27(4):5-8, November.

Hausman, K. (1993), U.S. psychiatrists' views on homosexuality differ from colleagues' in other countries. *Psychiatric News*, September 3.

Hausman, K. (1996), Gay psychiatrists break new ground internationally. *Psychiatric News*, p. 7, October 18. Retrieved March 29, 2002, from the American Psychiatric Association Web Site: <http://www.psych.org/pnews/96-10-18/wpa.html>.

Hausman, K. (2001), Finland's Parliament assesses U.S. reparative-therapy study. *Psychiatric News*, 36(24):11, December 21. Retrieved March 29, 2002, from <http://pn.psychiatryonline.org/cgi/content/full/36/24/11>.

Hettinga, N. F. (1998), International fears and national affairs: Same-sex marriage in the Netherlands. *Newsletter of the Association of Gay and Lesbian Psychiatrists*, 24(1):5-6, 9, January.

Hettinga N. F., Feijen R. A., Oele, B. L., Tuinebreijer, W., Van Ham, P. & Van Der Plaats, W. G. (1998), *Gay Psychiatrists: An Amsterdam Perspective*. Workshop conducted at the 151st Annual Meeting of the American Psychiatric Association, Toronto, Canada, May.

Hettinga N. F., Feijien R. A., Tuinebreijer, W., Oele, B. L. & Van der Plaats, W. G. (2001), *Narcissism Below Sea Level: A Dutch View of Future Gay Developments*. Workshop conducted at the 154th Annual Meeting of the American Psychiatric Association, New Orleans, LA, May.

Hire, R. O. (2001), An interview with Frank Rundle, MD. *J. Gay & Lesb. Psychother.*, 5:83-98.

Isay, R. (1989), *Being Homosexual: Gay Men and Their Development*. New York: Farrar, Straus and Giroux.

Junge, S. R. (1989), *Verschlüsselung von Homosexualität in Krankengeschichten? Die Position 302.0 (Homosexualität) der internationalen Krankeitenklassification (ICD) der Weltgesundheitsorganisation* [Encoding of homosexuality in the history of disease? The World Health Organization's listing 302.0 (Homosexuality) of the International Classification of Diseases]. In: *Homosexualität und Gesundheit [Homosexuality and Health]*, eds. U. Gooss & H. Gschwind. Berlin, Germany: Verlag Rosa Winkel, pp. 187-90.

Kjaer R. (2003), Look to Norway? Gay issues and mental health across the Atlantic Ocean. *J. Gay & Lesb. Psychother.*, 7(1/2):55-73.

Kjaer, R. & Selle, M. (2001), Letter to the Editor. *Newsletter of the Association of Gay and Lesbian Psychiatrists*, 27:15, April.

Klinger R. L. (1994), Psychiatric treatment of gay men and lesbians: overcoming homophobia. In: *Tolerance, Unity Amidst Diversity: The Role of Psychiatrists*, ed. E. Mercer. Amsterdam, Netherlands-Kiev, Ukraine: Geneva Initiative Network Publication, pp. 26-32.

Krajeski, J. P. (1996), Homosexuality and the Mental Health Professions: A Contemporary History. In: *Textbook of Homosexuality and Mental Health*, eds. R. P. Cabaj & T. S. Stein. Washington, DC: American Psychiatric Press, pp. 17-31.

Lee, K. (1995), *The Impact of Pacific Rim Culture on Gay and Lesbian Asians and Asian Americans.* Paper presented at the Seventh Scientific Meeting of the Pacific Rim College of Psychiatrists, Fukuoka, Japan.

Lee, S. (1996), Cultures in psychiatric nosology: The CCMD-2-R and classification of mental disorders. *Culture, Medicine, Psychiatry*, 20:421-72.

Lee, S. (2001), From diversity to unity: The classification of mental disorders in 21st-century China. *Psychiatry Clinics of North America*, 3:421-31.

Mental Disorder Redefined, Homosexuality Excluded (2001), *People's Daily*, March 12. Retrieved March 30, 2002 from the China Internet Information Center Web Site: <http://www.china.org.cn/english/9002.htm>.

Monroe, R. (1974), American Psychiatric Association Council Report, The Council on Research and Development. *Amer. J. Psychiat.*, 131:486-7.

Nakajima, G. A. (1995), Lesbians and gays no longer ill in Japan. *Newsletter of the Association of Gay and Lesbian Psychiatrists*, 21(4):8, December.

Nakajima, G. A. (1996), International visiting psychiatrists. *Newsletter of the Association of Gay and Lesbian Psychiatrists*, 22(4):11, December.

Nakajima G. A. (1999), International Committee column. *Newsletter of the Association of Gay and Lesbian Psychiatrists*, 25(4):13-14, November

Nakajima, G. A. (2001), International Committee column. *Newsletter of the Association of Gay and Lesbian Psychiatrists*, 27(2):18, April.

Nakajima, G. A., Chan, Y. H., Lee, K. (1996), Mental Health Issues for Gay and Lesbian Asian Americans. In: *Textbook of Homosexuality and Mental Health*, ed. R. P. Cabaj & T. S. Stein. Washington, DC: American Psychiatric Press, pp. 563-582.

Nakajima, G. A., Dannecker, S., Cochand, P., Jensen, O. E., Gloor, R. & Singy, P. (1998), *International Perspectives on Gay Psychiatry.* Workshop conducted at the 151st Annual Meeting of the American Psychiatric Association, Toronto, Canada, May.

Nakajima, G. A., Guss, J. R., Lee, S. & Drescher, J. (2000), *Sex, Drugs, and Homosexuality.* Symposium conducted at the International Jubilee Congress of the World Psychiatric Association, Paris, France, June.

OCCUR (Association for the Lesbian and Gay Movement) (1994), A Brief Report on Psychiatry. *Pamphlet for OCCUR New York Tour A Brief Report on Psychiatry.* Pamphlet for OCCUR New York Tour, pp. 18-19.

Olarte, S. W. (2001), American Psychiatric Association Council Report, The Council on National Affairs. *Amer. J. Psychiat.*, 158:338-348.

Roughton, R. (2003), The International Psychoanalytic Association and homosexuality. *J. Gay & Lesb. Psychother.*, 7(1/2):189-196.

Sacks, H. S. (1997), A rising tide lifts all boats? A Chinese paradigm. *Psychiatric News*, November 21. Retrieved March 30, 2002, from the American Psychiatric Association Web Site: <http://www.psych.org/pnews/97-11-21/sacks.html>.

Stakelbeck, F., Frank U. (2003), From Perversion to Sexual Identity. Concepts of Homosexuality and Treatment in Germany. *J. Gay & Lesb. Psychother.*, 7(1/2):23-46.

Summerhawk, B., McMahill, C. & McDonald, D., eds. (1998), *Queer Japan Personal Stories of Japanese Lesbians, Gays, Bisexuals and Transsexuals.* Norwich, VT: New Victoria Publishers.

Tasman, A. (2000), More on APA's election, update on international affairs. *Psychiatric News*, February 4. Retrieved March 30, 2002, from the American Psychiatric Association Web Site: <http://www.psych.org/pnews/00-02-04/pres2a.html>.

Velasco, I. H. (1996), *Varios manuales de Psiquiatría aún tratan a los gays de "enfermos"* [Various psychiatric manuals even treat gays as "sick"]. *El Mundo*, August 28.

Wah-Shan, C. (2000), *Tongzhi Politics of Same-Sex Eroticism in Chinese Societies.* Binghamton, NY: The Haworth Press, Inc.

World Congress of Psychiatry (1999), *Proceedings of the Eleventh World Congress of Psychiatry.* Hamburg, Germany, August.

World Health Organization (1977), *Manual of the International Statistical Classification of Diseases, Injuries, and Causes of Death, Ninth Revision (ICD-9).* Geneva, Switzerland: World Health Organization.

World Health Organization (1988), Extract from "Clinical Descriptions and Diagnostic Guidelines" to Chapter V (F) of International Classification of Diseases, Tenth Revision, "Mental Behavioural and Developmental Disorders." List of categories (April 1988 draft). *British J. Psychiat.*, 152 (Suppl. 1):44-50.

World Health Organization (1992a), *The ICD-10 Classification of Mental and Behavioural Disorders: Clinical Descriptions and Diagnostic Guidelines.* Geneva, Switzerland: World Health Organization.

World Health Organization (1992b), *International Statistical Classification of Diseases and Health Related Problems, Tenth Revision (ICD-10)* (Vol. 1). Geneva, Switzerland: World Health Organization.

World Psychiatric Association (2000), *World Psychiatric Association Manual of Procedures, Second Edition.* Retrieved March 29, 2002, from <http://www.wpanet.org/generalinfo/manual.html>.

World Psychiatric Association (2002), *Sectorial Activities–WPA meetings.* Retrieved March 29, 2002, from <http://www.wpanet.org/sectorial/meeting.html>.

Wu, J. (2003), From *"Long Yang"* and *"Dui Shi"* to Tongzhi: Homosexuality in China. *J. Gay & Lesb. Psychother.*, 7(1/2):117-143.

Yanhai, W. (1997), Homosexuality still an illness in China. *Newsletter of the Association of Gay and Lesbian Psychiatrists*, 23:4, November.

Yanhai, W. (2001), Becoming a gay activist in contemporary China. *J. Homosexuality*, 40:47-64.

APPENDIX

List of Relevant Psychiatry Organizations

Association of Gay and Lesbian Psychiatrists (AGLP)
4514 Chester Avenue
Philadelphia, PA 191143-3707
USA
Tel: 1 (215) 222-2800
Fax: 1 (215) 222-3881
e-mail: aglp@aglp.org
website: www.aglp.org
International Membership $60

Journal of Gay & Lesbian Psychotherapy
(Official journal of AGLP)
Editor-in-Chief: Jack Drescher, MD
For subscribing information contact:
The Haworth Press, Inc.
10 Alice Street
Binghamton, NY 13904-1580
USA
Tel: 1 (607) 722-5857
Tel: 1-800-429-6784 (toll free US and Canada)
Fax: 1-800-895-0582
e-mail: getinfo@haworthpressinc.com

American Psychiatric Association (APA)
1400 K Street, NW
Washington, DC 20005
USA
Tel: 1 (202) 682-6000
website: http://www.psych.org

APA Committee on Gay, Lesbian, and Bisexual Issues,
Tel: 1 (202) 682-6097

APA Commission on Global Psychiatry in the International Research Programs
in the *DSM* Programs of the Division of Research
Tel: 1 (202) 682-6855

APA International Membership and Annual Meeting-International Participants
Tel: 1 (202) 682-6128; http://www.psych.org/joinapa/internationalapp.pdf;
International Membership $150

Australasian Gay, Lesbian, and Bisexual Interest Group in Psychiatry (AGLBIG)
Dr. Graeme Croft, Chair, AGLBIG
Suite 6, 206 Albert Street
East Melbourne, Victoria, 3002
Australia
Tel: 61 3 94194591
e-mail: gracroft@ozemail.com.au
website: http://members.ozemail.com.au/~msa

Gay and Lesbian Mental Health Special Interest Group
Royal College of Psychiatrists
17 Belgrave Square
London SW1X P8G
United Kingdom
website: www.rcpsych.ac.uk/college/sig/gayles.htm

World Psychiatric Association, Secretariat
International Center for Mental Health,
Mount Sinai School of Medicine of New York University
Fifth Avenue and 100th Street, Box 1093
New York, NY 10029-6574
USA
Tel: 1 (718) 334-5094
e-mail: wpa@dti.net
website: http://www.wpanet.org

Section on Psychiatry and Human Sexuality:
Rubén Hernández-Serrano, MD, Chair

The International Psychoanalytical Association and Homosexuality

Ralph Roughton, MD

SUMMARY. With more than 10,000 members in 30 countries, the International Psychoanalytical Association (IPA) considers itself the world's primary psychoanalytic accrediting and regulatory body. Until 1998, however, the IPA had never addressed the problem of antihomosexual discrimination, even though gay people were excluded from most of its institutes and societies. Rationalizations for discrimination included: (1) "homosexuality is pathological and therefore disqualifying," (2) "as a scientific organization the IPA should avoid political issues," and (3) "because there is no written policy excluding homosexuals, there is no problem." Nevertheless, recent progress was finally made when an official nondiscrimination policy was adopted by the IPA. Homosexuality has become a topic for scientific programs and newsletter dialogue, but full implementation of the policy will require an ongoing process. This article presents the history of that process to date. *[Article copies available for a fee from The Haworth Document Delivery Service: 1-800-HAWORTH. E-mail address: <getinfo@haworthpressinc.com> Website: <http://www. HaworthPress.com> © 2003 by The Haworth Press, Inc. All rights reserved.]*

KEYWORDS. Antihomosexual bias, discrimination, gay and lesbian psychoanalysts, homosexuality, International Psychoanalytic Association, prejudice, psychoanalytic training, sexual orientation

Ralph Roughton is a Training and Supervising Analyst, Emory University Psychoanalytic Institute, and Clinical Professor of Psychiatry, Emory University Department of Psychiatry and Behavioral Sciences. He was a member of the International Psychoanalytical Association's House of Delegates, 1996-99.

[Haworth co-indexing entry note]: "The International Psychoanalytical Association and Homosexuality." Roughton, Ralph. Co-published simultaneously in *Journal of Gay & Lesbian Psychotherapy* (The Haworth Medical Press, an imprint of The Haworth Press, Inc.) Vol. 7, No. 1/2, 2003, pp. 189-196; and: *The Mental Health Professions and Homosexuality: International Perspectives* (ed: Vittorio Lingiardi, and Jack Drescher) The Haworth Medical Press, an imprint of The Haworth Press, Inc., 2003, pp. 189-196. Single or multiple copies of this article are available for a fee from The Haworth Document Delivery Service [1-800-HAWORTH, 9:00 a.m. - 5:00 p.m. (EST). E-mail address: getinfo@haworthpressinc.com].

With more than 10,000 members in 30 countries, the International Psychoanalytical Association (IPA) considers itself the world's primary psychoanalytic accrediting and regulatory body, working with component societies to provide standards of training and to develop educational and research programs (IPA, 2001). As such, this organization is in a position to influence attitudes and policies throughout the psychoanalytic world. And yet, prior to 1998, the subject of antihomosexual discrimination had been avoided, its existence denied.

Appointed to the IPA Program Committee, Richard Isay, MD had hoped to introduce changes similar to those he had begun initiating in the American Psychoanalytic Association (Isay, 1996). In an exchange of letters in 1992 with IPA President Joseph Sandler, Isay asked that the Executive Council (EC) sponsor a resolution on homosexuality and discrimination, similar to the one adopted by the American Psychoanalytic Association. Sandler expressed willingness to consider the matter; but, at two different meetings of the EC, he found that "we did not have time to discuss the proposal sufficiently," and therefore he suggested that Isay submit his proposal as a resolution at the next Business Meeting of the IPA. Isay responded that it was unlikely to get a majority vote in that setting, but hoped that the Council would find time to discuss it in the future (Isay, 1992; Sandler, 1992). It is uncertain if any further official discussion of this issue took place prior to 1999.

At the time of Isay's initiative, the IPA structure fostered the concentration of power in an elite, conservative group of analysts; this made it unlikely that a challenge to tradition could get a hearing. The arcane inner politics of the IPA may be of little interest to readers of the *Journal of Gay & Lesbian Psychotherapy*, but progress in overcoming antihomosexual discrimination is directly related to changes that made the IPA a more democratic organization. So a brief explanatory background seems necessary.

The IPA is divided into three regions: North America, Latin America, and Europe. The President, the Treasurer, and nine Vice-Presidents (three from each region) are elected by the worldwide membership and make up the governing Executive Council. In the early 1990s, in response to a growing movement toward more representative government, a 27-member House of Delegates was created. Each region elects its own nine members, assuring closer local involvement than the internationally elected Executive Council. Nevertheless, this body had little power, being conceived as only an advisory body to the EC. It could recommend but not enact changes.

In 1996 I was elected by the American Psychoanalytic Association (APsaA) to be one of nine North American representatives to the IPA House of Delegates. In electing an openly gay analyst with the stated goal of introducing a resolution to end antihomosexual discrimination in the IPA, the APsaA implicitly supported that effort, as did the other North American delegates when I presented it to them.

Another encouraging factor was that Otto Kernberg, MD had been elected and would take office as President in 1997. Although his early writings conflated homosexual orientation with psychopathology, I had heard that his views were changing and that he would likely oppose discriminatory practices.[1] I informed Kernberg of my intentions by letter and asked his advice on how to proceed. He recommended having it come up through a resolution in the House of Delegates, and he assured me that he would support it when it came to the EC for debate and vote.

I made the tactical decision not to bring this up in the House as "the new kid on the block" but to let the delegates from Europe and Latin American get to know me first as an individual, then as a gay man; then I would introduce what I knew would be a controversial issue. The House met twice a year and I had participated in two meetings by the time I was invited by the Program Committee to be a speaker on a Panel on Homosexuality at the 1997 IPA Congress in Barcelona. During this clinical presentation, I identified myself as an openly gay training analyst–virtually an oxymoron at that time. I think no other members of the House of Delegates attended that particular panel, or they would have seen some psychoanalysts displaying antihomosexual feelings in person, in the here and now.

I was dismayed that the first comment from the floor after my presentation was about homosexuals molesting young boys; I found out only later that the Barcelona newspapers that morning had been full of the latest pedophile scandal. Another speaker from the floor demanded to know, "What are we going to do when 'they' [gay analysts] come knocking on our doors wanting to join our analytic societies?" Granted that I spoke in English and he in Spanish, but there was simultaneous translation; so I didn't know whether he had understood that I was one of "them." Those were the worst responses, but altogether it did not feel like a friendly atmosphere. In addition, another gay colleague and I had put up a notice on the bulletin board, inviting other gay and lesbian participants to join us for drinks after the panel. Someone had written slurring graffiti on the notice.

On the positive side, this display of analysts' homophobia mobilized even stronger support from other North American members. Still, recoiling somewhat in anxious timidity, I waited a year before I opened the dialogue with other House members. I notified them by e-mail of my intentions, sent them some written materials about the problem internationally and about the changes that had been made in the APsaA, and asked that it be put on the agenda for our next meeting.

In December 1998, we had a preliminary discussion. Delegates took it seriously enough that we agreed to set aside two hours at our next meeting for further discussion. This meeting would take place during the summer of 1999 at the biennial IPA Congress in Santiago, Chile.

Discussion in the House of Delegates at that meeting lasted several hours and was cordial and respectful, even when there was significant disagreement. My original proposal was a statement only about discrimination based on sexual orientation. It became apparent that this would not pass, so it was modified as suggested by delegates from Canada to a broader nondiscrimination policy. The final wording was:

> The IPA opposes any discrimination against anyone on the basis of gender, ethnic origin, religious belief, or homosexual orientation. Selection of candidates for psychoanalytic training is to be made only on the basis of qualities directly concerned with the ability to learn and to function as a psychoanalyst. Further, it is expected that the same standard will be used in the appointment and promotion of members of educational faculties, including training and supervising analysts.

Opposition to this proposal came from two directions. In general, the Latin American delegates opposed the proposal based on the assumption that homosexuality is pathological and therefore disqualifies one for psychoanalytic training. Several of the delegates said they themselves did not hold this view but their members back home did. An interesting side issue is that, after several hours of discussion, we finally learned that, in Latin American countries, the term "sexual orientation" includes all the paraphilias or perversions. Therefore, it would be interpreted by them that we were wanting to protect analytic training for pedophiles and necrophiliacs as well homosexuals. That is the reason for using "homosexual orientation" rather than simply "sexual orientation."

The other opposing view, coming mostly from European delegates, was not based on assumptions about pathology but on a cultural difference in how they regard "identity politics." They considered it not a proper organizational issue but rather a matter of concern only for an individual's private life. In fact, some expressed the view that "naming a category" creates a problem and in fact limits individual freedom. They also felt that this was an American problem and did not concern them; they had no such problem.

The resolution was passed by a vote of 18 in favor, 1 opposed, and 5 abstaining. The strongest backing came from the North American delegates, but obviously there were some affirmative votes from the other regions as well. I do believe that my presence as a member of the group–known first as an individual who then identified himself as gay–made a difference in the eventual passage of this resolution. This experience reinforces the axiom that the most effective way to dispel prejudice is to get to know individuals as people rather than as stereotypes.

In addition, it was important that we presented this strictly as a matter of discrimination and justice and that we tried to avoid getting into controversies about origin, development, and psychopathology. We only need to know that it is possible to be both homosexual and a competent psychoanalyst, and this is demonstrably true. If that is true, then any rejection based solely on homosexual orientation is clearly discrimination. I believe it was also important in the passage of this resolution by the House of Delegates that we were able to present the positive experience with openly gay and lesbian candidates in North American psychoanalytic institutes since the adoption of a similar nondiscrimination policy in the APsaA.

I must hasten to emphasize, however, that passage by the House of Delegates was only a recommendation to the EC to adopt it as policy and incorporate it into the rules governing the IPA. What happened in the Executive Council was a different story. Not being a member of that group, I was not allowed to attend the meeting to present or discuss the resolution. It was carried to the EC by the three officially designated representatives from the House, only one of whom personally supported the resolution.

After hours of bitter debate in the EC, with opposition similar to that described in the House, only the North American delegates and one from England were in favor. Others strongly opposed any mention of sexual orientation at all. It was reported to me by more than one delegate present in the meeting that the immediate past president of the IPA, a man from Latin America, had made an impassioned statement that "homosexuality is an illness."

Finally the Executive Council passed a substitute resolution by a vote of 8 in favor, 5 opposed, and 1 abstaining. In a procedural twist, the 5 opposed were the North American and English delegates, who voted against this resolution because they wanted the stronger statement that named homosexual orientation. The final wording was:

> On the basis of its commitment to ethical and humanistic values, the IPA opposes any discrimination of any kind. Selection of candidates for psychoanalytic training is to be made on the basis of qualities concerned with the ability to learn and to function as a psychoanalyst. Further, it is expected that this same standard will be used in the appointment and promotion of members of educational faculties, including training and supervising analysts. (Minutes, Executive Council, July 1999)

The voting pattern suggested that the defeat was the result of the combination of two opposing viewpoints, but for different reasons: those who consider homosexuality pathological and those who opposed naming any categories.

This outcome was discouraging and dismaying, but it had the positive effect of arousing a spirited informal debate throughout the IPA meeting. And it gained us a strong supportive group far beyond the small original group who promoted the resolution. Many members were outraged that, in refusing to adopt a policy of nondiscrimination that specifically named homosexual orientation, the IPA seemed to be affirming a prejudicial stance of accommodation to those who regard it as pathological. It was even suggested that some European delegates' supposed idealistic reasons for opposing the stronger policy may have in fact been a cover for underlying antihomosexual prejudice.

Some members took the position that an inclusive nondiscrimination policy *was* adopted; others saw it as a subterfuge that seemed to be nondiscriminatory but which in fact would allow those who consider homosexuality pathological, to continue to reject gay candidates and faculty and to claim that they are not discriminating, but that those individuals are simply not qualified.

Some members of the House of Delegates were also angry that its strongly supported resolution was overturned by the Executive Council. It also raised procedural questions about two of its representatives to the EC voting against a resolution that had been passed by such a wide margin in the House.

For these many reasons, the controversy did not go quietly into the night. The House formally asked the EC to reconsider, and this forced it to be placed on the agenda for the next meeting in Nice in 2001. Again, the issues were debated and again the decision was to leave the policy as it was adopted in 1999.

The outrage among members of the APsaA was intensified, and it erupted in a spontaneous dialogue on this organization's Internet Openline discussion. The discussion went on for weeks and was led not by gay members, but by supportive gay-friendly colleagues. Some even questioned the ethical position of our remaining members of the IPA when it adopted a policy that violated the APsaA's own nondiscrimination position.

Meanwhile, the editor of the IPA newsletter, Alex Holder, had asked me to write an article for its Dialogue series. The issue was delayed and did not appear until after the Nice meeting (Roughton, 2001a). Five analysts from different regions had been invited to write a discussion of my paper, and then my response to them appeared in December (Roughton, 2001b).

In addition, the officers of the APsaA made a formal protest to the new President of the IPA, Daniel Widlocher from Paris. In a letter they asked him to forthrightly address discrimination issues in the IPA; and both they and I requested that the president clarify whether the IPA policy, which supposedly opposes any form of discrimination, does in fact include homosexual individuals.

On September 21, 2001, Dr. Widlocher responded in a letter to me, which was subsequently printed in the newsletter: "I can state unequivocally on behalf of the Council of the IPA that homosexual orientation is included within this resolution" (2001, p. 4).

The Executive Committee of the APsaA then drafted a resolution to include this specific clarification in the formal policy statement. It was to be brought up at the next meeting of the IPA Executive Council in January 2002. Dr. Widlocher asked, however, that the IPA Executive Committee be allowed to introduce it as their resolution, which would give it greater clout.

At the January meeting, the issues were again discussed. The new resolution now had the strong backing, not only of the House of Delegates but also the officers of the APsaA and the IPA. In addition, the composition of the EC had been changed by a new election. Only one of the voting members in the July 2001 decision in Nice was still a voting member of this Council. Whether this was a more accepting group is unknown, but at least they were not in the position of wanting to defend their previous vote.

The discussion was rigorous and lasted about two hours. The most vocal opposition came from one delegate who wanted to have some scientific evidence that homosexuals are capable of functioning as psychoanalysts. This was effectively countered by North American Vice President Robert Pyles, who pointed out that this evidence does exist in the experience of the American Psychoanalytic Association. However, he also said that, even taking her argument at face value, it would make more sense to ask for evidence that homosexuals are *not* capable of functioning as psychoanalysts before we take away rights and privileges for an entire group. This apparently had a big impact on the thinking of the delegates (Robert Pyles, personal communication). By an "almost unanimous vote," the policy was amended to read:

> On the basis of its commitment to ethical and humanistic values, the IPA opposes any discrimination of any kind. This includes, but is not limited to, any discrimination on the basis of age, race, gender, ethnic origin, religious belief or homosexual orientation. Selection of candidates for psychoanalytic training is to be made only on the basis of qualities directly concerned with the ability to learn and to function as a psychoanalyst. Further, it is expected that this same standard will be used in the appointment and promotion of members of educational faculties, including training and supervising analysts. (Minutes, IPA Executive Council, January 2002)

This is a very significant event in the life of international psychoanalysis. I have been told privately by some European colleagues that their analytic societies were waiting to see what the IPA did and that they would follow in their own policy. This is not the end of the story, obviously. There will continue to be overt opposition from those who strongly disagree, and their will be more widespread covert resistance to change, stemming both from conscious and unconscious beliefs and prejudices.

But it is a major progressive step. I also believe that it is a lesson in group process in an organization where multiple diversities of language, culture, and theory tend to divide us. Begun by a small group of gay analysts who were determined to bring about change, the cause was then taken up by our heterosexual colleagues, who were outraged for us by the prejudice and injustice and were also outraged by the need for organization and political reform. Once justice has been established, then it will be time to explore all the interesting scientific questions about sexuality, both homosexual and heterosexual.

NOTE

1. Editor's Note: See Kernberg, O. F. (2002), Unresolved issues in the psychoanalytic theory of homosexuality and bisexuality. *J. Gay & Lesb. Psychother.*, 6(1):9-27.

REFERENCES

International Psychoanalytical Association (1999), *Minutes of the Executive Council*, July.

International Psychoanalytical Association (2001), *Membership Handbook*.

Isay, R. (1992), Unpublished letters to Joseph Sandler, June 1 and August 12.

Isay, R. (1996), *Becoming Gay: The Journey to Self-Acceptance*. New York: Pantheon.

Roughton, R. (2001a), Dialogue: Homosexuality: Clinical and technical issues. *International Psychoanalysis*, 10(1):17-26.

Roughton, R. (2001b). Dialogue: Homosexuality: Continued. *International Psychoanalysis*, 10(2):29-32.

Sandler, J. (1992). Unpublished letter to Richard Isay, August 6.

Widlocher, D. (2001), Letter to Ralph Roughton, September 21, 2001. *International Psychoanalysis*, 10(2):4.

On Fritz Morgenthaler, MD (1919-1984):
An Interview with Paul Parin, MD

Luisa Mantovani, PhD

The late Fritz Morgenthaler, MD, as noted in several of the European papers in this collection, was an early pioneer in psychoanalytic theorizing about homosexuality from a nonpathological perspective. I met with Dr. Morgenthaler's colleague and friend, Dr. Paul Parin, for the *Journal of Gay & Lesbian Psychotherapy* to discuss Parin's own work and that of Morgenthaler. Dr. Parin has also written on the subject of homosexuality in a paper entitled, "The Mark of Oppression."

Dr. Parin was interviewed in Zurich on a cold and windy afternoon in late January of 2002 in his apartment in a fascinating old building on the river of Lake Zurich. His home is full of souvenirs of his trips to Africa, as well as paintings by Fritz Morgenthaler. Dr. Parin, who is 85 years old, had recently lost his wife. He spoke openly for several hours, providing a fountain of wonderful memories of his life with his wife and friends, and particularly memories of his friend Fritz Morgenthaler.

Journal of Gay & Lesbian Psychotherapy: Could you tell me about your own educational background and training?

Dr. Parin: I was born in Slovenia, the son of Jewish family, a Swiss citizen. I began medical studies there but moved to Zurich in 1938 before the *Anschluss*

Luisa Mantovani is Psychotherapist and Psychoanalyst, Psicoterapia e Scienze Umane and in private practice, Bologna, Italy.

The author wishes to thank Paul Moor of Berlin for his assistance in translating the references.

[Haworth co-indexing entry note]: "On Fritz Morgenthaler, MD (1919-1984): An Interview with Paul Parin, MD." Mantovani, Luisa. Co-published simultaneously in *Journal of Gay & Lesbian Psychotherapy* (The Haworth Medical Press, an imprint of The Haworth Press, Inc.) Vol. 7, No. 1/2, 2003, pp. 197-206; and: *The Mental Health Professions and Homosexuality: International Perspectives* (ed: Vittorio Lingiardi, and Jack Drescher) The Haworth Medical Press, an imprint of The Haworth Press, Inc., 2003, pp. 197-206. Single or multiple copies of this article are available for a fee from The Haworth Document Delivery Service [1-800-HAWORTH, 9:00 a.m. - 5:00 p.m. (EST). E-mail address: getinfo@haworthpressinc.com].

10.1300/J236v07n01_12

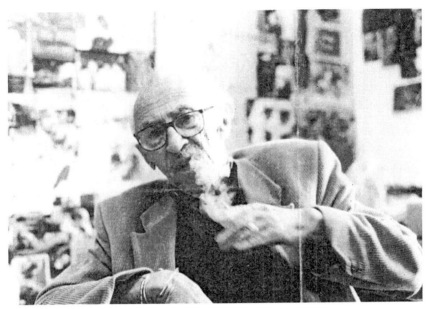

Paul Parin, MD, in Zurich (2002)

of Austria to finish medical training. When German troops occupied Yugoslavia in 1941, the rest of my family fled and settled in Switzerland. In the beginning, I worked as a neurologist in the Neurological Clinic of Zurich. I was very interested in psychoanalysis, but in Zurich after the war there were only three psychoanalysts. I did my training with Professor Rudolf Brun.

JGLP: How did you come to know and work with Fritz Morgenthaler? Could you talk about Morgenthaler's education and training?

Dr. Parin: Morgenthaler was born in 1919. He was the son of a famous painter, Ernst Morgenthaler. He attended primary school in Paris and high school and medical school in Zurich where he got his medical degree in 1945. The first time I met Morgenthaler was in 1946 in Prijedor, Yugoslavia, where he was working in a hospital with Goldy Matthèy, who would later become my wife. They were both working with a Swiss, postwar relief agency. Morgenthaler became very ill at the time with pneumonia and I treated him, giving him the first injection of penicillin in my medical career. After Yugoslavia, Morgenthaler worked in Paris as an assistant in cardiology until 1951.

He returned to Zurich in 1952 where he would become a psychoanalyst. From 1958 onward, he founded and directed "The Psychoanalytic Seminar of Zurich" for many years. This was a joint enterprise with the Swiss Society of

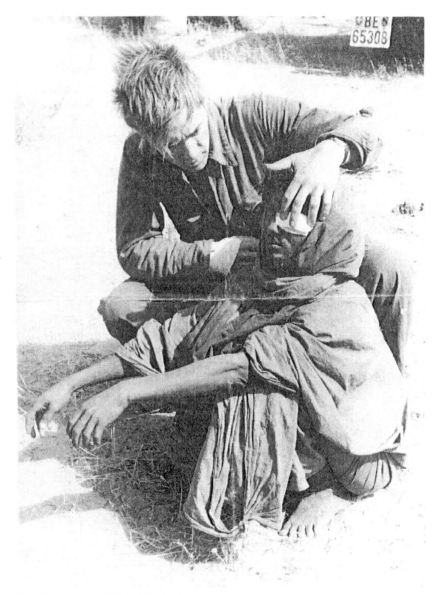

Fritz Morgenthaler, MD, in Mauritania (1971)

Psychoanalysis (SSP), an affiliate of the International Psycho-analytic Association. After 1977, the SSP would no longer recognize the Psychoanalytic Seminar, but Morgenthaler was always faithful to it. He was editor of the Bulletin of the Seminar and Director of Education and Training. In the 1960s, he became a member of the sponsoring committee for Italy. He taught psychoanalysis in many institutes, particularly in Italy, including Bologna, Milano, Torino, Parma, and Bari. His seminars on dreams were very famous.

Between 1954 to 1971, my wife, Goldy Parin-Matthèy, and I traveled six times to West Africa with Morgenthaler to do scientific studies of ethnopsychoanalysis. Morgenthaler made another important scientific trip in 1979-80 to Papua-New Guinea with the ethnologists Florence Weiss and Milan Stanek as well as with Morgenthaler's own son, Marco, an anthropologist. Before and after these years Morgenthaler traveled extensively with his wife Ruth in India, China, Australia, Indonesia, and South and Central America.

Morgenthaler, before attending university, was a professional juggler; he was always ready for the show. Not only had he mastered this art in his youth, he practiced it until he was old. In addition to being a physician and a psychoanalyst, Morgenthaler was also an artist and a painter. In the last 15 years of his life, he dedicated himself to painting, both before and during his journeys and then later in his studios in Sardinia, Bologna and Zurich. He had about 12 exhibitions of his watercolors and oil paintings in Basel, Zurich, and Berlin and became quite famous as painter. He died of a stroke while in Ethiopia in 1984.

JGLP: Do you know how Morgenthaler first came to write and theorize about the subject of homosexuality?

Dr. Parin: His interest in sexual problems, and particularly in male homosexuality came out of his work with homosexual patients and because he himself had homosexual relations. Although Morgenthaler was married and had two sons, during his marriage he had numerous relations with men. He never hid these relations, although he also never exhibited them either.

JGLP: Could you explain Morgenthaler's theory of homosexuality and how it differed from mainstream psychoanalytic theories of his time? How does Morgenthaler's writing about homosexuality fit into his wider contributions to the field of psychoanalysis?

Dr. Parin: Morgenthaler's work can be understood within two contexts. First, for psychoanalysts up to Morgenthaler's time, male homosexuals were problematic patients. They were particularly resistant to the treatment, and it was presumed that homosexual patients, without exception, had serious and early developmental disturbances. The second context is that Morgenthaler writes critically of traditional psychoanalytic theories of homosexuality from *within* Freudian traditions. I will try to summarize some of the most important points:

1. Psychoanalysis discovered infantile sexuality as the expression of the polymorphous perverse, sexual predisposition of man. However, psychoanalysis cannot refer solely to infantile sexuality in order to explain mature sexual behavior; for there is no linear correlation between infantile sexual instinctual impulses and adult sexual modes of expression and experience.[1]

2. There exists a normal development toward homosexuality just as there exists a normal development toward heterosexuality. Morgenthaler delineated, within the context of the transferential relationship a framework for the "development toward homosexuality." He recognized three decisive stages in this development to which I refer you to his well-known article on homosexuality.

3. Where one finds neurotic disturbances of homosexual individuals, they have to be considered within the context of *their* normal phases of development, just as the neurotic disturbances of heterosexuals have to be thought about in relationship to their specific development.

4. The "sexual" is distinguishable from "sexuality." The "sexual" is linked to the id. The id is without aim, timeless, without a precise direction and equivalent to the "emotional." It is movement; it is expressed in love, in creativity, in every form of human relationships, and also, naturally, in psychoanalysis between the two participants. The "sexual," simply put, is "there" from the beginning; it does not develop, it cannot be modified nor become ill.[2]

5. In contrast to the "sexual," an individual's "sexuality" results from development, in the course of which the emotional movements of the id come under the control of the ego. Therefore, one's "sexuality" can develop and conform to various modes. Under the influence of the external environment and of the super-ego which shape it, "sexuality" can be modified in different ways; it can be modified or deformed; it can lead to frustrating or satisfying experiences, or cause happiness. Only in "sexuality," either when it is developing or when it is already formed, does one find an object, a direction, or a goal. "Sexuality" can become ill and it can be cured. In the treatment of sexual disturbances, it is necessary to attenuate or eliminate the dictatorship of "sexuality" on the "sexual" and to restore the free expression of the "emotional," of the "sexual."

6. Not only do adolescent experience leave their imprint on any form of sexuality, they can also inflict or unleash regressive or compensatory developments, in the sense of a secondary "neuroticization."

From these new concepts of Morgenthaler, which I've tried to review, one arrives at a new orientation, not only in doing therapy but also in the conceptualization of sexual behavior. Human sexuality is not imaginable without development. Therefore, to ask whether homosexuality is either innate or acquired means to pose the question in an incorrect manner. Any sexuality–homosexuality, heterosexuality, or perversions of any type–can, but not necessarily be troubled, deformed, or made ill by developmental conflicts. However, the "sexual" can never be considered ill.

JGLP: I believe Morgenthaler first published on the subject of homosexuality in 1975. Do you recall the initial reactions to his work on homosexuality when it was first published?

Dr. Parin: I don't remember particular reactions. I think that was because the changed cultural climate in the Western world after the Second World War was more open to sexuality, even if that climate was inclined to newer forms of repression and manipulation. I know that Morgenthaler's book "Homosexuality Heterosexuality Perversion," was translated in English in 1988, after his death and it was published by The Analytic Press. I have no idea how it was sold or accepted in the United States.

JGLP: As you probably know, in 1973 the American Psychiatric Association removed homosexuality as a disorder from its *Diagnostic and Statistical Manual.* Did Swiss psychiatrist use this diagnosis?

Dr. Parin: The directors of the Swiss schools of psychiatry were so conservative that the didn't treat homosexuality as an illness, they simply ignored it.

JGLP: Are you aware if there has been greater acceptance of gay and lesbian mental health professional into the Swiss psychoanalytic community?

Dr. Parin: In the Swiss Psychoanalytic Society, there were no struggles about homosexuality. I never heard a word or a gossip about homosexuality and particularly not about Morgenthaler's homosexuality. It never came up. Instead, they had other prejudices. For example, they accused our group, the Psychoanalytic Seminar, of being too political, too leftist or of being paid by Moscow to destroy psychoanalysis.

JGLP: You have written about homosexuality yourself. What was the nature of the dialogue between you and Morgenthaler on the subject?

Dr. Parin: Morgenthaler didn't speak very much about his patients, but sometimes he did. I knew his ideas long before they were published. He had no lesbian patients. Generally they went to female analysts and there were more female analysts in that time in Zurich than male analysts. We had no practical or theoretical differences, only Morgenthaler's idea that there is no bisexuality. This was a kind of theoretical construction he made. But he himself was the typical bisexual.

I agree with him in distinguishing the "sexual" from "sexuality." He said, "yes there is sexuality, and it may be neurotic. However, the sexual is an emotion, it is in art, in love, in sexual feelings." This the original idea of Freud's libido. Morgenthaler came back to the libido. At least, this is what I understood.

More or less we have the same ideas, but Morgenthaler had a kind of abstract thinking about psychoanalysis. I personally never had supervision with him. When I needed supervision, I went to another colleague because Morgenthaler's explanations were so theoretical. He was so abstract that you had to translate what he said in practical terms again. He was very complicated. For example, when his friend Heinz Kohut–and they were good friends– came to Europe, he came to visit us in Sardinia where Morgenthaler had a house. I said to Morgenthaler, "This man is so cold. I don't like him." And Morgenthaler said something like, "It is very simple: If you understand that he takes you as a self-object and that he rejects the object, you take five or six steps to establish this relationship, and then you can become friends with him." It was very complicated!

Morgenthaler was gifted with a uniquely suitable background which allowed him to creatively–and without prejudice–think about sexuality and his empirical experiences in new ways. He was the son of upper class parents and raised in a family of artists. As he was not from the average bourgeois family, he was relatively free of certain restrictions of class and caste. Through exposure to the life of artists, he found a subculture that made playful relating to the body a professional aim. In the course of his many travels, he expanded upon his basic criticism of social relationships, thanks in particular to his ethno-psychoanalytic experiences.

I'll give two examples. Among the Dogon of Mali, no behavior–even sexual ones–is considered indecent, as long as the behavior isn't hidden. Only that which is hidden, covered up, or separated from society is taboo. Among the Iatmul (a district of Sepik in Papua-New Guinea), public and ritual transvestitism is used in the service of social integration,[3] to bring the generations together and to construct sexual identities.[4]

But I return overall to Morgenthaler's artistic gifts, the unique freedom he had to concern himself with sexual phenomena upon which he based his theoretical and clinical work. In his rapport with form and colors, in his ability to give form to his own emotions, he expressed a vital sentiment which allowed him to access the "sexual" in every form.

NOTES

1. Editor's Note: The American ego-psychologist, Heinz Hartmann, made a related point in 1960, criticizing the "genetic fallacy–the equation of a behavior with its origins, or the assumption that a behavior originating out of conflict is inevitably linked to conflictual difficulties" (p. 58). In parallel with Morgenthaler, although from an Inter-

personal psychoanalytic perspective, this point was further taken up by Stephen A. Mitchell in one of his two seminal papers on homosexuality (1981). See Hartmann, H. (1960), *Psychoanalysis and Moral Values*. New York: International Universities Press and Mitchell, S. A. (1981), The psychoanalytic treatment of homosexuality: Some technical considerations. *Internat. Rev. Psycho-Anal.*, 8:63-80.

2. Editor's Note: In Werner Muensterberger's introduction to the English translation of Morgenthaler's book, he notes that the latter "approaches sexuality from a nonconflictual angle, simply presupposing a natural condition of inner harmony. In terms of his hypothesis, ego development and libido organization are powerfully influenced by the prevailing cultural ethos. It is this unequivocal position that leads him to new, persuasive psychoanalytic insights and alternative criteria for distinguishing between the 'normal' and the 'perverse'" (p. xi-xii).

3. Editor's Note: See Bateson, G. (1936), *Naven*. Cambridge: Cambridge University Press.

4. The following is from Werner Muensterberger's introduction to Morgenthaler's book: "Morgenthaler applies his newly won insights about such practices in discussing his treatment of a brilliant writer whose developmental conflicts led him to transvestitism and passive homosexual encounters. The analyst, after having conducted field research among the Iatmul, revised his point of view vis-à-vis this man's state of mind. Recognizing his own ethnocentric prejudice, he was led to reinterpret the particular variables that entered into his patient's leanings. In the case of the people of New Guinea, ritualized transvestitism served as a sensory mode of reinforcing body ego and body identity. And Morgenthaler discovered that his Swiss patient's obsessional dressing in female garments fulfilled the same function. It was the man's way to adapt, in a primary-process fashion, his illusionary creative achievement to the conditions of his environment. What the Iatmul dramatize in their transvestite ceremonies this patient attempted to act out in his, to us, perverse impersonation" (p. xi).

SELECTED BIBLIOGRAPHY OF FRITZ MORGENTHALER

Morgenthaler, F. (1951a), *Übertragungs und Widerstandmechanismen in der Psychoanalyse* [Transference and mechanisms of resistance in psychoanalysis]. *Schweizer Zeitschrift für Psychologie*, 10(2):116-135.

Morgenthaler, F. (1951b), *Darstellung einer Analyse* [Portrayal of an analysis]. *Schweizer Zeitschrift für Psychologie*, 10(3):185-200.

Morgenthaler, F. (1952a), *Mischneurose und psychosomatische Krankheit. Die doppelt geführte Reaktionsbildug* [Mixed neurosis and psychosomatic illness: Doubly led reaction formation]. *Schweizer Zeitschrift für Psychologie*, 11(1):33-45.

Morgenthaler, F. (1952b), *Père et fils. Analyse d'un cas clinique* [Father and son: Analysis of a clinical case]. *Psyché*, 65/66/67.

Morgenthaler, F. (1961), *Psychoanalytische Technik bei Homosexualität* [Psychoanalytic technique in the instance of homosexuality]. *Jahrbuch für Psychoanalyse*, 2:174-198.

Morgenthaler, F. (1966), Psychodynamic aspects of defence with comments on technique in the treatment of obsessional neuroses. *Int. J. Psychoanal.*, 47:204-209.

Morgenthaler, F. (1969a), *Aspekte der Anwendung der Psychoanalyse* [Aspects of the application of psychoanalysis]. *Jahrbuch der Psychoanalyse*, 6:9-18.

Morgenthaler, F. (1969b), *Störungen der männlichen und weiblichen Identität in der psychoanalytischen Praxis* [Disorders of masculine and feminine identity in psychoanalytic practice]. *Psyche*, 26:58-77.

Morgenthaler, F. (1974), *Die Stellung der Perversionen in Metapsychologie und Technik* [The place of perversions in metapsychology and technique]. *Psyche*, 28:1077-1098.

Morgenthaler, F. (1975), Reflex-modernization in tribal societies. In: *Shelter, Sign and Symbol*, ed. P. Oliver. New York: Overlook Press.

Morgenthaler, F. (1977), Traffic forms of perversion and the perversion of traffic forms. *Kursbuch*, 49.

Morgenthaler, F. (1979), *Innere und äußere Autonomie* [Internal and external autonomy]. *Neue Züricher Zeitung*, 7/8 July.

Morgenthaler, F. (1980a), *Homosexualität* [Homosexuality.] *Berliner Schwulenzeitung* [Berlin Gay Newspaper].

Morgenthaler, F. (1980b), *Homosexualität*. In: *Therapie sexueller Störungen [Therapy of Sexual Disorders]*, ed. V. Sigusch, Second edition. Stuttgart & New York: Georg Thieme Verlag.

Morgenthaler, F. (1983), *Psychoanalyse und Sexualität* [Psychoanalysis and sexuality]. In: *Sexualtheorie und Sexualpolitik [Sexual Theory and Sexual Politics]*, ed. V. Sigusch. Stuttgart.

Morgenthaler, F. (1984), *Homosexualität. Heterosexualität. Perversion*. Frankfurt/M/Paris: Qumran. Translated as *Homosexuality Heterosexuality Perversion*, trans. A. Aebi. Hillsdale, NJ: The Analytic Press, 1988.

Morgenthaler, F. (1986), *Der Traum. Fragmente Zur Theorie und Technik der Traumdeutung [The Dream: Fragments on the Theory and Technique of Dream Analysis]*, eds. P. Parin, G. Parin-Matthèy, M. Erdheim, R. Binswanger & Hans-Jürgen Heinrichs. Frankfurt & New York.

SELECTED ETHNOPSYCHOANALYTIC COLLABORATIONS

Parin, P., Morgenthaler, F. & Parin-Matthèy, G. (1956/57), *Charakteranalytischer Deutungsversuch am Verhalten >primitiver< Afrikaner* [A character-analytic attempt to interpret behavior of "primitive" Africans]. *Psyche*, 10.

Parin, P., Morgenthaler, F. & Parin-Matthèy, G. (1965a), *Formen der Übertragung bei Westafrikanern* [Forms of transference with West Africans]. *Schweizer Zeitschrift für Psychologie*, 24(4).

Parin, P., Morgenthaler, F. & Parin-Matthèy, G. (1968), *Aspekte des Gruppenich. Katamnese bei den Dogon* [Aspects of the group ego: Katamnesis with the Dogon]. *Schweizer Zeitschrift für Psychologie*, 27(2).

Parin, P., Morgenthaler, F. & Parin-Matthèy, G. (1969), *Ist die Verinnerlichung der Aggression für die soziale Anpassung notwendig?* [Is internalization of aggression necessary for social adjustment?]. In: *Bis hierhin und nicht weiter [Thus Far and No Farther]*, ed. A. Mitscherlich. Munich.

Parin, P., Morgenthaler, F. & Parin-Matthèy, G. (1971), *Fürchte deinen Nächsten wie dich selbst. Psychoanalyse und Gesellschaft am Modell der Agni in Westafrika* [*Fear Thy Neighbor as Thyself: Psychoanalysis and Society on the Model of the Agni in West Africa*]. Frankfurt: Suhrkamp.

Parin, P., Morgenthaler, F. & Parin-Matthèy, G. (1975), *La méthode psychanalitique au service de la recherche ethnologique* [The psychoanalytic method in the service of ethnological research]. *Connexions*, 15.

Parin, P., Morgenthaler, F. & Parin-Matthèy, G. (1982), *Unsere Vorstellungen von normal und anormal sind nicht auf andere Kulturen übertragbar* [Our conceptions of normal and abnormal are not transferable to other cultures]. In: *Das Fremde verstehen* [*Understanding the Unfamiliar*], ed. H.-J. Heinrichs. Frankfurt/M.

Index

ABVA (AIDS *Bhedbhav Virodhi*
        Andolan), 101n,151-152,153
Achté, Kalle, 79,83,87n,88n
Acquired immunodeficiency syndrome
        (AIDS)
    in China, 129,130,131,132,134
    in Germany, 31,40
    in India, 151-152
Adolescents
    gay, 64-65
    homosexuality development in, 31
Adoption, by same-sex couples, 59
Age of consent
    in Germany, 26,41n
    in the United Kingdom, 8,17
AGLP. *See* Association of Gay and
        Lesbian Psychiatrists
AIDS. *See* Acquired
        immunodeficiency syndrome
AIDS *Bhedbhav Virodhi Andolan*
        (ABVA), 101n,151-152,153
AIZHI Newsletter, 130,133
Akbarbadi, Nazeen, 149
American Medical Association, 177
American Psychiatric Association, 60
    annual meetings, AGLP activities
        at, 176-178
    Caucus of Gay, Lesbian, and
        Bisexual members, 166
    Commission on Global Affairs, 176
    Commission on Global Psychiatry,
        166-167
    Committee on Gay, Lesbian, and
        Bisexual Issues, 106,166,167,
        168,178-179

Council of International Affairs,
        175
    description of, 166-167
    Fact Sheet: Gay, Lesbian, and
        Bisexual Issues, 174
    gay and lesbian members, 195
    International Affairs Office,
        167-168,169,170
    members' attitudes towards sexual
        orientation change, 110-111n
    Office of International Affairs,
        167-168
    position on gay and lesbian
        psychoanalysts, 66
    statement about reparative and
        sexual conversion therapies,
        65
    statements and resolutions about
        homosexuality, 106,107,167,
        178-179,181-182n,190
    support for depathologization of
        homosexuality in China, 134
American Psychoanalytic Association,
        position on homosexuality,
        106
American Psychological Association,
        position on depathologization
        of homosexuality, 134
Anal intercourse, 100,148-149,153-154
Anang Rang (Kalyanmalla), 160n
Andersson, Claes, 80,81,82
Anima/animus, 17
Antidiscrimination laws

10.1300/J236v07n01_13

SPECIAL 25%-OFF DISCOUNT!

Order a copy of this book with this form or online at:
http://www.haworthpressinc.com/store/product.asp?sku=
Use Sale Code BOF25 in the online bookshop to receive 25% off!

The Mental Health Professions and Homosexuality
International Perspectives

____ in softbound at $18.71 (regularly $24.95) (ISBN: 0-7890-2059-9)
____ in hardbound at $37.46 (regularly $49.95) (ISBN: 0-7890-2058-0)

COST OF BOOKS _____	☐ **BILL ME LATER:** ($5 service charge will be added)
Outside USA/ Canada/	(Bill-me option is good on US/Canada/
Mexico: Add 20% _____	Mexico orders only; not good to jobbers,
POSTAGE & HANDLING _____	wholesalers, or subscription agencies.)
(US: $4.00 for first book & $1.50	☐ **Signature** _____
for each additional book)	
Outside US: $5.00 for first book	☐ **Payment Enclosed: $** _____
& $2.00 for each additional book)	☐ **PLEASE CHARGE TO MY CREDIT CARD:**
SUBTOTAL _____	☐Visa ☐MasterCard ☐AmEx ☐Discover
in Canada: add 7% GST _____	☐Diner's Club ☐Eurocard ☐JCB
STATE TAX _____	**Account #** _____
(NY, OH, & MIN residents please	
add appropriate local sales tax	**Exp Date** _____
FINAL TOTAL _____	**Signature** _____
(if paying in Canadian funds, convert	(Prices in US dollars and subject to
using the current exchange rate,	change without notice.)
UNESCO coupons welcome)	

PLEASE PRINT ALL INFORMATION OR ATTACH YOUR BUSINESS CARD

Name
Address
City   State/Province   Zip/Postal Code
Country
Tel   Fax
E-Mail

May we use your e-mail address for confirmations and other types of information? ☐Yes ☐No
We appreciate receiving your e-mail address and fax number. Haworth would like to e-mail or
fax special discount offers to you, as a preferred customer. **We will never share, rent, or
exhange your e-mail address or fax number.** We regard such actions as an invasion of
your privacy.

Order From Your Local Bookstore or Directly From
The Haworth Press, Inc.
10 Alice Street, Binghamton, New York 13904-1580 • USA
Call Our toll-free number (1-800-429-6784) / Outside US/Canada: (607) 722-5857
Fax: 1-800-895-0582 / Outside US/Canada: (607) 771-0012
E-Mail your order to us: Orders@haworthpress.com

Please Photocopy this form for your personal use.
www.HaworthPress.com

BOF03